LEARN YOGA
IN A WEEKEND

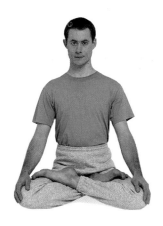

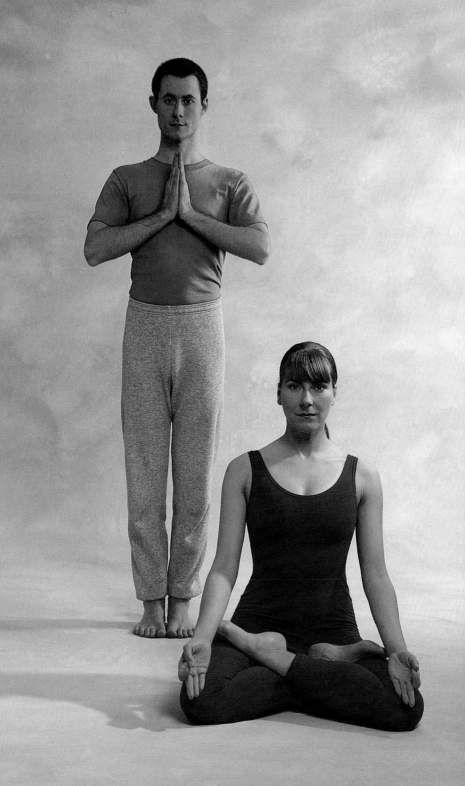

LEARN YOGA
IN A WEEKEND

THE SIVANANDA YOGA VEDANTA CENTER

Photography by Jane Stockman

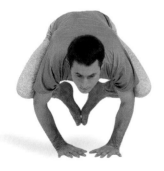

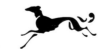

ALFRED A. KNOPF
New York
1993

A DORLING KINDERSLEY BOOK

This edition is a Borzoi book published in 1993 by Alfred A. Knopf, Inc., by arrangement with Dorling Kindersley.

Designer Sam Grimmer
Project Editor Sarah Larter
Editor Katie John
Senior Art Editor Amanda Lunn
Series Editors Jo Weeks, Laura Harper
Deputy Art Director Tina Vaughan
Deputy Editorial Director Jane Laing
Production Controller Helen Creeke

Library of Congress Cataloging-in-Publication Data

Sivananda Yoga Vedanta Center (London, England)
  Learn yoga in a weekend / by Sivananda Yoga Vedanta Center. -- 1st American ed.
      p. cm. -- (Learn in a weekend series)
      Includes index.
      ISBN 0-679-42751-1
      1. Yoga, Hatha. I. Title.
RA781.7.S576 1993
      613.7'046--dc20   93-721
                                                          CIP

Computer page make-up by Cloud 9 Designs
Reproduced by Colourscan, Singapore
Printed and bound by Arnoldo Mondadori, Verona, Italy

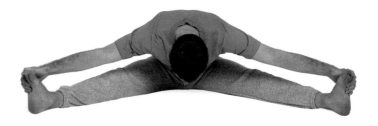

CONTENTS

·

Introduction 6

PREPARING FOR THE WEEKEND 8

What is yoga? 10
Space & clothes 12
You & your body.................. 14
Strong & supple.....................16
Proper breathing..................18
The sequence of asanas 22

THE WEEKEND COURSE 24

Day 1

Opening a session................26
The Sun Salutation 28
Leg raises 32
The Headstand................... 34
The shoulder cycle..............38
The Fish.............................44
Bend & straighten 46
Sitting poses........................48

Day 2

Stretching back....................50
Back bends..........................54
Joint mobility 58
Spinal twisting 60
Balancing poses....................62
Standing asanas...................66
Final relaxation 72

AFTER THE WEEKEND 74

Organizing your practice 76
Advanced asanas..................78
Good food...........................80
Meditation 82
Health & life 84
Yoga for all 86
Yoga & sport 88
Where to practice................90

Glossary 92
Index 94
Getting in touch 96
Acknowledgments 96

INTRODUCTION

·

ON BEHALF OF the International Sivananda Yoga **Vedanta** Centers, we offer *Learn Yoga In A Weekend* as an inspirational guide to anyone interested in learning about this ancient discipline and enhancing the quality of their lives. The techniques covered in this book were not invented by the Sivananda Yoga Centers, but are historical methods that have been adapted for modern lifestyles by our teacher Swami Vishnu-devananda. Yoga cannot be learned by simply understanding its theory; for it to work, you must put this theory into practice. Although it is not possible to master all the techniques of yoga in a weekend, you can utilize even this short amount of time to begin learning the **asanas**, and use them as a foundation for further development. We think that the step-by-step

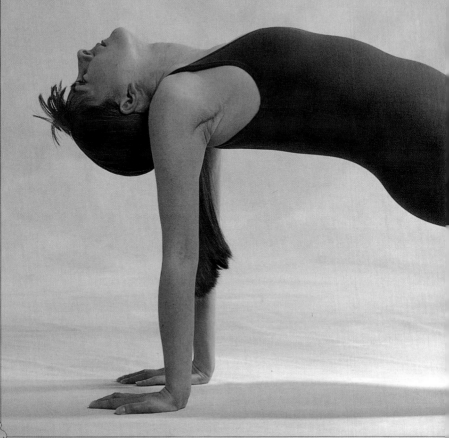

instructions set out in this book will get you off to a good start. The most effective way to learn yoga is to do a little at a time, and keep to a regular practice schedule. Please be careful not to go beyond your capacity; do not try to work too quickly or too intensively. Although you may wish to learn at home, initially it may be more beneficial to have lessons or take a course with a group, as the collective energy will sustain and inspire you.

Our best wishes are with you.

SWAMI SARADANANDA

PREPARING FOR THE WEEKEND

Getting ready for your weekend of yoga

———————— • ————————

A YOGA WEEKEND IS AN ADVENTURE of disciplined self-discovery. The exercises, or **asanas**, will unlock tensed muscles, rejuvenate your heart, and restore flexibility to your joints and ligaments. Set aside a quiet time, when you will not be disturbed, for the sessions. If you are at home, you might even want to take the telephone off the hook or put the answering machine on so that you are not distracted. You may practice yoga at any time of the day, but make sure that you have not eaten for several hours, as it is best to do the exercises on an empty stomach. For this reason, many yoga students prefer to practice first thing in the morning. Try to do the asanas in a relaxed manner; do not move abruptly, or you may pull a muscle. Yoga is not a competitive sport; the

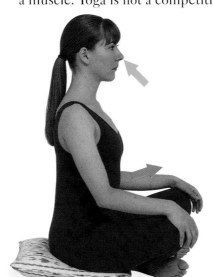

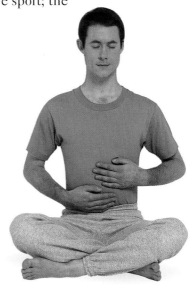

ESSENTIAL EXERCISES
Breathing exercises are an essential part of yoga practice. These techniques, which are known as **pranayama**, will clear your lungs, and will help to recharge your physical and mental energy levels (see pp.20-21).

UNDERSTANDING BREATHING
In order to perform the breathing exercises and the **asanas** correctly, you must begin by understanding how your lungs work. This knowledge will enable you to make use of their full capacity (see pp.18-19).

purpose is to keep you as fit, flexible, and peaceful as possible. Never practice on a bed or soft mattress. A single blanket folded in half or quarters will cushion your body, yet still give you the firm support of the ground. Always wear loose, comfortable clothing, and remember to remove glasses, contact lenses, and jewelry before you begin. During the yoga session, breathe through your nose rather than your mouth, and try to keep your mind focused on your breath. Do not try to go beyond your body's capability.

*Throughout the book you will notice terms printed in **bold** type; these words are defined in the glossary (see pp.92-93).*

TESTING YOUR STRENGTH

Each body has its good points and limitations. Most of us are strong in some ways and supple in others. Factors such as the time of day also make a difference; your muscles are always stiffer in the morning, as they are hardly used while you are asleep. Before you start this course, test the strength and flexibility of each muscle (see pp.16-17).

STRETCH AND CONTRACT

The action of each muscle is determined by its line of pull, which is unique to it. If you know where your major muscle groups are, and in which direction they move, you will be able to exercise them more effectively during your yoga sessions (see pp.14-15).

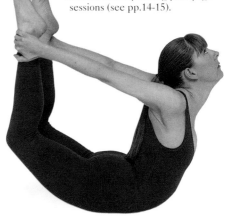

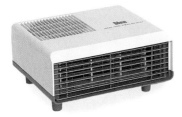

PROPER EQUIPMENT

Warm, comfortable surroundings are vital for yoga sessions. Your clothes need not be specially bought, but they must allow your body to move freely (see pp.12-13).

WHAT IS YOGA?

Explaining the origins and principles of yoga

THE WORD **YOGA** MEANS "UNION". Yoga is the practical aspect of a philosophy called **Vedanta**, which is set out in the **Upanishads** and maintains that there is one absolute reality that underlies everything in the universe. Yoga techniques have been practiced for over 5,000 years. Among the most important teachings of yoga philosophy are instructions on how to put the body under the control of the mind. The Indian sage, Patanjali, defined yoga as being achieved through methods such as controlling the breath and holding the body in steady poses. These techniques are known as **hatha yoga**.

THE FIVE PRINCIPLES

In order for a car to function properly, it requires five things: a lubricating system, a battery, a cooling system, fuel, and an intelligent driver to steer and control it. Your body has similar requirements; the Five Principles of yoga were developed by Swami Vishnu-devananda to fulfil them.

PROPER BREATHING
The breath links your body to its battery, the **solar plexus**, where potential energy is stored. The breathing techniques of **pranayama** release this energy for physical and mental rejuvenation.

• FEET
Starting with your feet and moving upward, consciously relax every muscle and joint in your body.

PROPER RELAXATION
Relaxation acts as the body's cooling system. When your body and mind are overworked, their efficiency decreases. Proper Relaxation recharges them, releases all tension, and allows you to make the most of your energy.

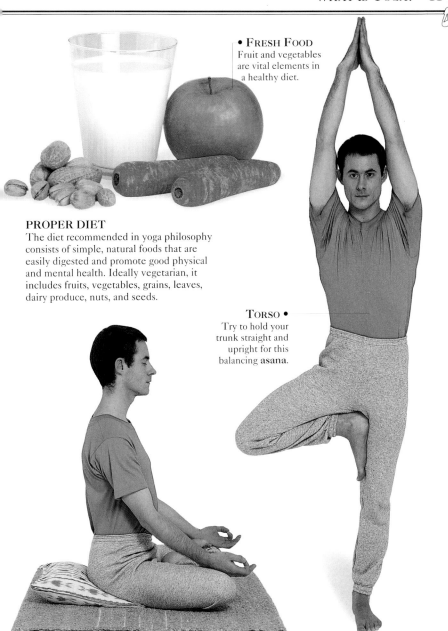

• FRESH FOOD
Fruit and vegetables
are vital elements in
a healthy diet.

PROPER DIET
The diet recommended in yoga philosophy
consists of simple, natural foods that are
easily digested and promote good physical
and mental health. Ideally vegetarian, it
includes fruits, vegetables, grains, leaves,
dairy produce, nuts, and seeds.

TORSO •
Try to hold your
trunk straight and
upright for this
balancing **asana**.

THOUGHT AND MEDITATION
Positive Thought and **Meditation** enable you
to become a good "driver". Positive Thought
purifies your intellect and gives you conscious
control over your instincts. Meditation puts
you in touch with your innermost being.

PROPER EXERCISE
In yoga this takes the form of **asanas**. These
"lubricate" your body, improving circulation
and flexibility. Asanas are unlike the violent
movements in most other types of exercise,
which may actually worsen fatigue.

Space & Clothes

Creating a comfortable environment for your yoga sessions

·

You will need a minimum of equipment to begin your practice of yoga. It is the ideal method of exercise to learn at home. You may choose to practice inside or, when the weather is fine, you may prefer to do your yoga session in the fresh air. If you are outdoors, find a location that is relaxing and secluded enough for you to practice undisturbed. For yoga you do not need to buy expensive, specially designed clothing. Dress simply and comfortably – try a leotard or loose-fitting exercise clothes, so that your movements are not constricted and you are not too hot or too cold.

A Place to Practice

For practicing indoors, you will need a clear space with no furniture. The room should be comfortably heated and well ventilated. It is important to choose a place that is free from disturbances and distractions. If the room has no carpet, a rug or a folded blanket can be placed on the floor.

Cushions •
You may want to sit on a cushion during **meditation** and for the breathing and preliminary exercises.

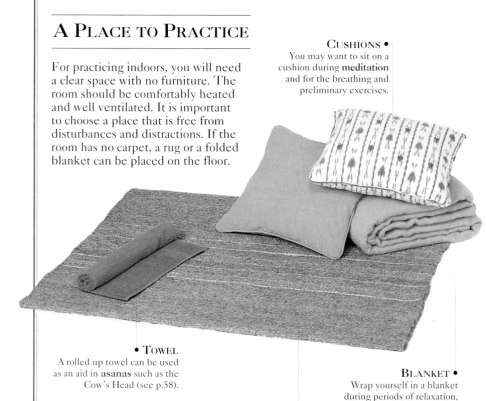

• Towel
A rolled up towel can be used as an aid in **asanas** such as the Cow's Head (see p.58).

Rug •
A rug can be placed on the ground if you do not have a carpet covering the floor.

Blanket •
Wrap yourself in a blanket during periods of relaxation, as your body temperature will drop while you are resting.

WHAT TO WEAR

You do not need any special clothing for yoga, but what you wear must be comfortable and allow the maximum range of movement. It is best to wear items made from natural materials. If you have long hair tie it back, so that it does not interfere with your **asanas**. Keep a sweater to hand in case you start to feel cold.

T-SHIRT •
A loose-fitting cotton T-shirt is ideal wear for yoga sessions.

TROUSERS •
Comfortable tracksuit bottoms or trousers are suitable and inexpensive.

LEOTARD •
A leotard is not essential, but it will allow you freedom of movement. Choose one made from a stretch cotton mix.

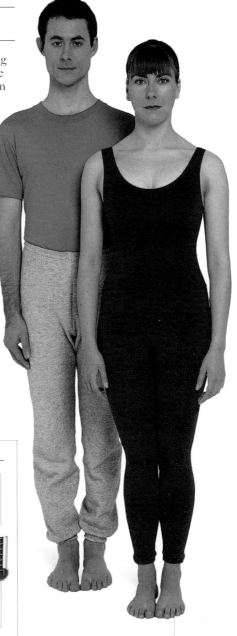

WARMTH

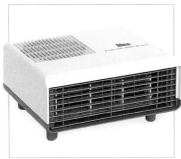

Keeping warm during a session is essential. A small electric heater can help to keep the room in which you practice at a comfortable temperature.

• FEET
Do not wear shoes for yoga, as they will restrict your foot movements. Bare feet are preferable, but if you are cold you can wear socks.

YOU & YOUR BODY

Understanding how your body works and is constructed

BEFORE YOU EMBARK on your yoga course, it is wise to become familiar with your physical make-up. The body is a remarkable machine, consisting of a strong skeletal structure supported by flexible muscles and ligaments. Your muscles have a dual role: they hold you steady when you are in a particular position, and by extending and flexing they allow you to move your body. In order to work most efficiently, they must be long enough to permit the free movement of your joints, as well as short and strong enough to provide postural stability. Yoga **asanas** exercise your body naturally, stretching each of its muscles slowly and taking into account its limitations and capabilities. Regular yoga practice enables you to use your joints to the full, enhances flexibility in your limbs and spine, and results in the correct alignment of your skeletal frame.

MOVEMENT

The cycle of **asanas** (see pp.22-23) is designed to contract and extend your muscle groups in the right order. To tone your muscles, you flex certain groups fully while letting the opposite muscle groups extend as far as possible.

EXTENSION
Muscles need to be able to stretch, to allow free movement. The Forward Bend shown here fully extends the hamstrings and the back muscles.

• SPINE
The vertebrae from the **lumbar** to the **cervical** region of the spine are stretched in this pose.

• ABDOMEN
As the muscles of the spine flex in the Bow, their opposites, the abdominals, are extended.

CONTRACTION
In this pose, the muscles extended in the Forward Bend are contracted, stretching the opposing group of muscles in the abdomen.

KNOW YOUR BODY

Stress, poor posture, and spending too long sitting or standing can all put a strain on your body. If you know your basic anatomy, you will be able to focus on problem areas, and so derive the most benefit from your **asanas**.

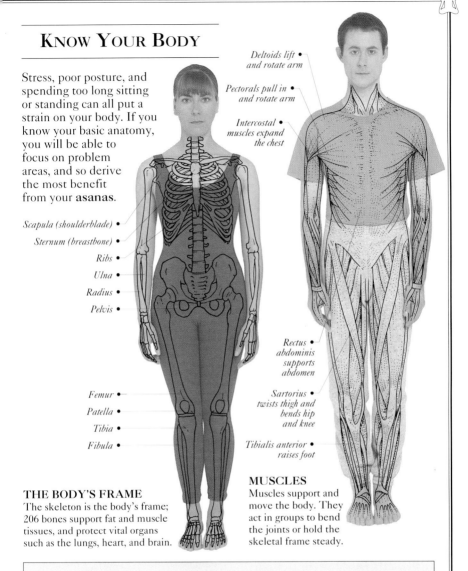

Deltoids lift and rotate arm •

Pectorals pull in and rotate arm •

Intercostal muscles expand the chest •

Scapula (shoulderblade) •
Sternum (breastbone) •
Ribs •
Ulna •
Radius •
Pelvis •

Rectus abdominis supports abdomen •

Femur •
Patella •
Tibia •
Fibula •

Sartorius twists thigh and bends hip and knee •

Tibialis anterior raises foot •

THE BODY'S FRAME
The skeleton is the body's frame; 206 bones support fat and muscle tissues, and protect vital organs such as the lungs, heart, and brain.

MUSCLES
Muscles support and move the body. They act in groups to bend the joints or hold the skeletal frame steady.

YOGA & YOU

Yoga is for everyone, young and old. It is different from other forms of exercise in that yoga **asanas** are intended to bring about a harmonious balance in your body and your mind. While there is no one who should be categorically exempted from doing yoga exercises, consult your doctor before beginning a course if you suffer from any medical condition or if you have any doubts. This book is designed as an introduction to the classical teachings of yoga; if you wish to learn more about this discipline, and to attempt more difficult asanas, it is best to work with a qualified teacher. If the exercises shown in the course are practiced in the right spirit, they can be of great benefit to both mind and body. Remember, however, that yoga alone is in no way meant to be used as a medical prescription for any condition.

STRONG & SUPPLE

Tests to determine your muscular strength and flexibility

A HEALTHY BODY is both flexible and strong. The object of yoga is to balance suppleness with strength; regular practice allows these qualities to be maintained. Although none of us can avoid becoming less mobile as we grow older, poor posture and lack of exercise often hasten the process. For example, sitting hunched over desks or steering wheels for too long can cause tension in your back muscles and rounding of your chest and shoulders. The following tests will help you to locate areas of weakness and stiffness in your body.

MUSCLE STRENGTH

Your muscles must be strong enough to keep your body stable when you are standing or in any other pose. If they are weak, you will suffer from bad posture and limited joint movement. Using the information provided by the following tests, you can focus on **asanas** that will strengthen particular areas of weakness in your body.

OFF THE GROUND
This exercise tests your upper abdominal muscles. Lie on your front, with a partner holding your feet so that they do not lift off the floor. Then bend your arms up, arch your back, and raise your body as high as possible.

PELVIS •
Arch your spine upward from your pelvis.

• **FEET**
Lift your feet as high as possible.

LIFT YOUR LEGS
Lie on your back. Try to lift both legs so that they are at 90° to your body, while keeping your **lumbar** area flat. Any arching of your back indicates weakness in your abdominal muscles.

MUSCLE FLEXIBILITY

Muscles must be long enough to allow free joint movement. The following tests will reveal any limited joint motion. During your yoga sessions, gently try to stretch tight muscles. Do not attempt to compensate for stiffness by overstretching your more flexible muscles.

LEGS UP STRAIGHT
Lie on your back, and let a friend lift one of your legs as high as possible. Keep both legs straight. If your hamstring is tight, your leg will not rise far. Tight **lumbar** muscles will make your back arch.

HIPS •
Bend forward from your hips.

LEGS •
Keep your legs straight but relax your muscles.

TOUCH YOUR TOES
Sit with your spine and legs straight, then lean forward and try to touch your toes. This exercise will help you to feel the length of your back muscles, your hamstrings, and the muscles at the back of your calves.

BEND YOUR SPINE
Lie face down with your arms by your sides. Keeping your legs straight, ask a friend to lift your feet as high as possible. This exercise shows up stiffness in your back and in the muscles at the front of your chest.

PROPER BREATHING

Understanding and enhancing your breathing capability

TO LIVE IS TO BREATHE. Without oxygen, no cell in your body would be able to live for more than a few minutes. Most people use only a fraction of their full breathing capacity. This inefficiency allows fatigue and stress to set in. Proper breathing can tone up your entire system and enhance health and vitality. **Pranayama** breathing exercises are the link between the physical and mental disciplines of yoga. In all these exercises exhalation, rather than inhalation, is accentuated. This is because correct exhalation cleanses the lungs and speeds the elimination of toxins from your body.

BREATH AWARENESS

Understanding the mechanics of your lungs

THE MECHANICS

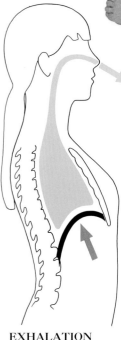

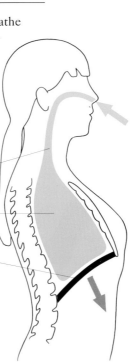

During yoga **asanas**, you breathe through your nose. When you inhale, your **diaphragm** moves downward and air is drawn into your lungs via your trachea and bronchial tubes. When you exhale, your diaphragm moves upward and pushes the air out of your lungs.

TRACHEA •
Air is drawn down your trachea to the lungs.

LUNGS •
Your lungs are protected within your ribcage.

DIAPHRAGM •
This provides 75% of the movement in respiration.

INHALATION
Your intercostal muscles and **diaphragm** stretch, and this pulls air into your lungs.

EXHALATION
As the **diaphragm** moves upward again, the air is pushed out of the lungs.

LYING DOWN

The following exercises teach you to breathe efficiently. Lie flat on your back. Put one hand on your abdomen. Breathe slowly and gently; feel your abdomen rise as you inhale and fall as you exhale. Keep your breathing slow, deep, and relaxed. This movement is important, as it brings air to the lowest and largest portion of your lungs.

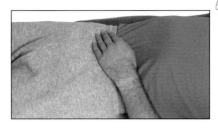

USING YOUR DIAPHRAGM
Deep abdominal breathing exercises the **diaphragm**. Proper use of this muscle can greatly enhance your breathing capacity.

• LEGS
Your legs are relaxed, as is the rest of your body.

• HAND
Rest one hand on your abdomen, and feel it move as you breathe.

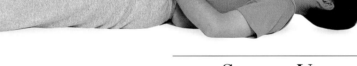

SITTING UP

HEAD •
Your head is erect and in line with your body.

Sit up straight, placing one hand on your abdomen and the other on your lower ribcage. Imagine that you can see your lungs. First, draw air into the lowest part of your lungs. Next, pull air into the middle of your lungs by stretching your intercostal muscles. Finally, feel the upper portion of your lungs expand. Most people breathe too shallowly, using only the upper part of their lungs; this practice is known as clavicular breathing, and ideally should be avoided.

• RIBCAGE
If you lay one hand on your ribcage, you will feel it expand as your muscles stretch it.

• ABDOMEN
As your lungs start to fill with air, feel your abdomen expanding.

BREATHING EXERCISES

*An introduction to **pranayama** – yoga breathing*

SINGLE NOSTRIL

Close your right nostril with your right thumb. Exhale completely through the left. Inhale to a count of 4, then exhale to a count of 8. Repeat 5 times. Close your left nostril with your ring and little fingers. Breathe through your right nostril, using the method given above. Repeat 5 times.

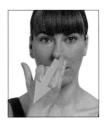

MUDRA
For **Vishnu Mudra**, extend your thumb, ring finger, and little finger, and fold down your other 2 fingers.

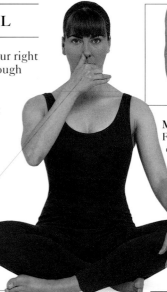

RIGHT HAND •
Your right hand assumes **Vishnu Mudra**.

LEGS •
Your legs are crossed in the **Easy Pose**, and your back is straight.

– *CUSHION COMFORT* –

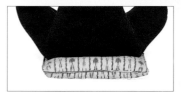

To keep a comfortable, straight pose, sit with a cushion under your buttocks when performing **pranayama**.

START TO ALTERNATE

When you are comfortable with Single Nostril Breathing, try breathing with alternate nostrils, as shown below, for a few rounds. Next, inhale with one nostril, but this time exhale with the other. Start a round by inhaling with the left nostril. Close it with your hand, then exhale right. Inhale right, close your right nostril, and exhale left. Do 10 of these rounds daily.

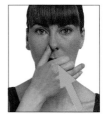

1. INHALE
Inhale with your left nostril to a count of 4.

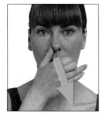

2. EXHALE
Exhale through this nostril to a count of 8.

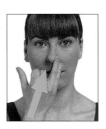

3. INHALE
Inhale with your right nostril to a count of 4.

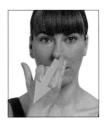

4. EXHALE
Exhale through this nostril to a count of 8.

ALTERNATE NOSTRIL

When you are comfortable with the preliminaries, begin full Alternate Nostril Breathing. Holding your right hand in **Vishnu Mudra**, close your right nostril with your thumb. Exhale fully through the left, then go through 1 round as shown. Try to perform at least 10 rounds daily for best results.

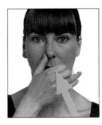
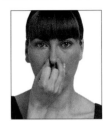

1. INHALE
Inhale with your left nostril to a count of 4.

2. RETAIN
Close both nostrils; hold to a count of 16.

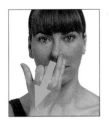
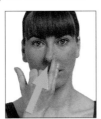
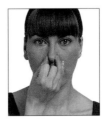
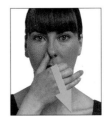

3. EXHALE
Exhale through the right, to a count of 8.

4. INHALE
Inhale through the right, to a count of 4.

5. RETAIN
Again, close nostrils for a count of 16.

6. EXHALE
Exhale through the left, to a count of 8.

KAPALABHATI

Kapalabhati, which means "shining skull", is believed to give the face an inner radiance. Sit cross-legged. Relax by taking a few deep breaths. Inhale deeply, then follow the steps below. Do 25 rapid pumpings in each round, and relax between rounds with a few deep breaths. Try to do at least 3 rounds before going on to the **asanas**.

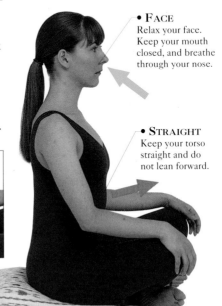

• **FACE**
Relax your face. Keep your mouth closed, and breathe through your nose.

• **STRAIGHT**
Keep your torso straight and do not lean forward.

1. AIR OUT
Pull in your abdominal muscles forcefully, as though you have been punched in the belly. Your **diaphragm** will move up quickly, and this will push the air out of your lungs.

2. AIR IN
To take in air, relax your abdominal muscles and let your **diaphragm** descend. Do not force the inhalation.

THE SEQUENCE OF ASANAS

Introducing the yoga **asanas**

SHOWN HERE IS THE sequence of **asanas** covered in the Weekend Course. Each asana or cycle of asanas prepares the body for the next pose. To derive the maximum benefit from this course, it is suggested that you do the sequence in the order specified here. The first pose taught is the Headstand, the "king of asanas". Next come the forward bends and their counterposes. These exercises are followed by the backward bends. The session ends with the lateral stretches and standing poses. Following the full program will balance, tone, and strengthen your entire body.

The Headstand (pp.34-37)

The Shoulderstand (pp.38-39)

The Plough (p.40)

THE HEADSTAND
One of the most famous poses, this is the first full **asana** taught during the Weekend Course.

SHOULDER POSES
In the Shoulder cycle, your spine is bent forward. The Fish, which follows, bends your spine backward.

The Fish (pp.42-43)

FORWARD BENDING
This seated pose stretches your upper body forward. It also extends the muscles in the backs of your legs.

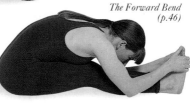

The Forward Bend (p.46)

BACK BENDS

After bending forward you move on to the backward bends. Each vertebra is given a stretch in these vital **asanas**.

The Cobra
(pp.50-51)

The Locust
(pp.56-57)

The Bow
(pp.54-55)

SPINAL TWISTS

After stretching your spine backward and forward, you give it a lateral twist in this **asana**.

The Spinal Twist
(pp.60-61)

The Crow
(pp.62-63)

BALANCING POSES

The Crow improves your concentration and strengthens your forearms.

Hands-to-Feet
(p.66)

STANDING

The Hands-to-Feet and the Triangle, in the standing cycle, work every part of your body.

The Triangle
(pp.67-69)

THE WEEKEND COURSE

Introducing your weekend yoga course

•

YOUR WEEKEND COURSE HAS fifteen skills spread over two days. On the first day, you are introduced to the warm-ups and the inverted and sitting poses. Day two involves reviewing the **asanas** learned in the previous day, then going on to the remaining poses. The skills are presented in the correct order, so you may wish to try part of each on day one. If you feel that covering all these poses in two days is too much for you, build up your practice more slowly. Try not to strain yourself, and do not omit the relaxation periods.

The Butterfly (pp.48-49)

DAY 1		*Minutes*	*Page*
SKILL 1	Opening a session	20	26-27
SKILL 2	The Sun Salutation	20	28-31
SKILL 3	Leg raises	10	32-33
SKILL 4	The Headstand	10	34-37
SKILL 5	The Shoulder cycle	20	38-43
SKILL 6	The Fish	10	44-45
SKILL 7	Bend & straighten	10	46-47
SKILL 8	Sitting poses	20	48-49

The Shoulderstand (pp.38-39)

KEY TO SYMBOLS

CLOCKS
Each skill is accompanied by an image of a clock. This shows the approximate time needed to assimilate and attempt the skill. The time is measured in minutes; blue sections indicate the number of minutes that have been allocated to the skill, and grey sections show you how much time has already been used on the course. The times given are only guidelines, though, and you may need to spend more or less time than suggested on a particular **asana**.

••••• RATING SYSTEM
All the skills are given ratings, to show the degree of difficulty involved. These ratings are indicated using bullets. One (•) denotes a straightforward skill that may be easily attempted by a beginner. Skills that are given five bullets (•••••) may be more complex, and you could require more practice before you attempt them. Some of the skills are divided into more than one pose; where this is the case, ratings are supplied for each **asana** in addition to the skill as a whole.

*Final relaxation
(pp.72-73)*

*The Sun
Salutation
(pp.28-31)*

DAY 2		Minutes	Page
SKILL 9	Stretching back	20	50-53
SKILL 10	Back bends	25	54-57
SKILL 11	Joint mobility	15	58-59
SKILL 12	Spinal twisting	10	60-61
SKILL 13	Balancing poses	15	62-65
SKILL 14	Standing asanas	20	66-71
SKILL 15	Final relaxation	15	72-73

*Triangle variations
(pp.68-69)*

*Hands-to-Feet
(pp.66-67)*

SKILL

1

OPENING A SESSION

Definition: *Mental and physical preparation for your session*

TO ENSURE THAT MAXIMUM BENEFIT is obtained from **asanas**, rest in the **Corpse Pose** for at least five minutes before proceeding with a session. In between asanas it is essential that you relax, breathing deeply, so the Corpse is also held for a short time between poses, and for longer at the end of each session (see pp.72-73). At the start of a session you also perform shoulder, neck, and eye exercises in the **Easy Pose**, a sitting posture that supports your back.

OBJECTIVE: Complete relaxation. *Rating* •

THE CORPSE POSE

Lie on your back and close your eyes. Shake out your shoulders. Turn your head from side to side, then return it to the center. Stay still, and take 10 deep breaths. Focus on your breath so that it becomes very gentle, with a slow and regular rhythm. Your heart rate will also slow to its resting level.

• **ARMS**
Place your arms so that they are at a 45° angle to your body.

• **BREATHING**
Breathe using your abdomen. Feel it rise with each inhalation, and sink with each exhalation.

FACE •
Remember to relax your face and keep your eyes closed.

• **FEET**
Place your feet 2ft (60cm) apart, so that your toes fall out.

FINGERS •
Let your fingers curl slightly. Keep your hands relaxed, with your palms upward.

HEAD •
Sit straight,
keeping your
head, neck,
and trunk
aligned.

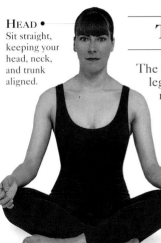

THE EASY POSE

The **Easy Pose** is a simple cross-
legged position, often adopted
naturally when sitting on the
floor. In yoga, it is one of the
basic positions used during
meditation, breathing, and
warm-ups. Sit upright and
keep your spine straight
so that it gives your
body firm support.

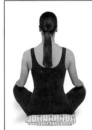

FOR COMFORT
Sitting on a cushion
keeps you straight
and eases pressure
on your knees.

• HANDS
Place your hands so that
they rest on your knees.

NECK ROLLS

Practice each set of neck rolls 3 times,
returning your head to the center
between exercises. Sit in the **Easy
Pose**. In the first exercise, bend your
neck forward slowly, hold for a few
moments, then bend it back. In the
second, tilt your head right, hold, then
tilt it left. In the third, look over your
right shoulder, hold, then look over
your left. Finally, rotate your head.

HEAD •
Rotate your
head clockwise
3 times and then
counterclockwise
3 times.

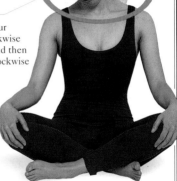

EXERCISING YOUR EYES

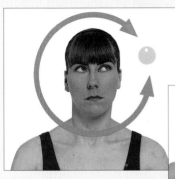

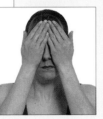

• Move only your eyes in these exercises.
Relax them in between. Unless another
number is specified, do each 10 times.
• To begin, look up and then look down.
• Open your eyes wide. Look from right
to left, then from left to right, and finish
by looking diagonally.
• Move your eyes in
circles. Start slowly,
and increase speed. Do
this movement 5 times
in each direction.
• Close your eyes. Rub
your hands together so
that they feel warm.
Cup them over your
eyes for 30 seconds.

Making circles (above). Palming (right)

2

THE SUN SALUTATION

Definition: *A twelve-part warm-up exercise*

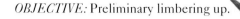

PERFORMED AT THE START of every **asana** session, each of the 12 positions of The Sun Salutation brings a different **vertebral** movement to your spinal column. Initially, just learn the physical movements. Once you have mastered these, tune them to your breathing. Do not start a session without doing this sequence.

OBJECTIVE: Preliminary limbering up.   *Rating •*

— Steps 1 & 2 —
STANDING

From the starting pose, below, exhale as you put your palms together at chest level. This first stance, called the Prayer Pose, centers your body. Next, inhale as you stretch your arms over your head and arch your back into the second position. Your hips come forward, and your head tilts back.

ARMS •
Keep your elbows straight, and align your arms with your ears.

KNEES •
Keep your knees straight, but do not lock them.

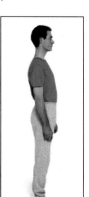

STARTING
Stand straight. Bring your feet together and hold your arms by your sides. Take a deep breath, and begin the Sun Salutation.

FEET •
Place your feet together. Balance your body weight evenly on them.

Steps 3 & 4
OVER & OUT

HEAD •
Stretch your head
right back and
look upward.

Exhale as you stretch forward
and down into the third position.
Place your hands on the ground
so that your fingers and toes
form a straight line. Bend your
knees if necessary, but keep
your hips held high. To assume
the fourth position, inhale as you
stretch your right leg back and
bend your knee to the ground.

• FOREHEAD
Tuck your forehead
in to your knees.

FEET •
Keep your feet
close together.

• HANDS
Keep your hands on the ground
on either side of your feet.

Steps 5 & 6
FACING THE FLOOR

For position 5, hold your breath as you
bring your left foot back next to your
right. Your body will be in a press-up
position. Try to align your head with
your neck and back, so that your spine
is straight. Exhale into position 6,
lowering your knees to the floor and
laying your chest down
between your hands.

HIPS •
Take care not
to drop or raise
your hips.

ELBOWS •
Keep your elbows straight when
you are in the press-up position.

KNEES •
Allow your knees to
touch the ground.

HIPS •
Your hips are
raised up off
the ground.

FOREHEAD •
Your head is tilted so that your
forehead touches the floor.

SKILL
2

— Steps 7 & 8 —

BACK & FORWARD

For position 7, inhale as you slide forward and lower your hips. Arch your chest and lean your head back. Exhale into position 8. Put your feet flat on the floor and lift your body into an "Inverted-V".

SHOULDERS •
Your shoulders are back and relaxed.

ARMS •
Bend your arms slightly and bring them in to your body.

• **ELBOWS**
Straighten your elbows when you come into this position.

• **HANDS**
Maintain the flat hand position of the previous step.

• **HEELS**
Stretch your heels toward the ground.

— Steps 9 & 10 —

COMING TO A CLOSE

Position 9 is a mirror image of the fourth position. Inhale, moving your right foot forward. Keep your left knee down, and look up. Next, exhale into position 10; put both feet together, stretch your hips up, and tuck your head in.

• **HIPS**
Keep your hips stretching up.

KNEE •
Drop your back knee to the ground.

FINGERS •
Your fingers remain in line with your toes.

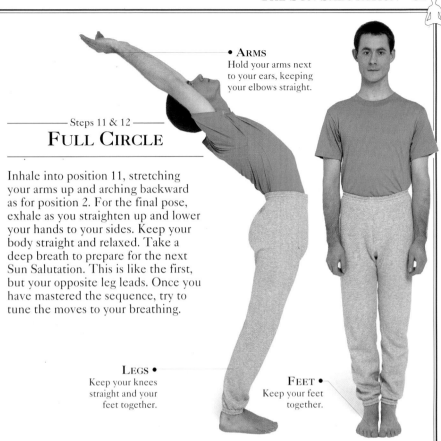

• ARMS
Hold your arms next
to your ears, keeping
your elbows straight.

—— Steps 11 & 12 ——
FULL CIRCLE

Inhale into position 11, stretching
your arms up and arching backward
as for position 2. For the final pose,
exhale as you straighten up and lower
your hands to your sides. Keep your
body straight and relaxed. Take a
deep breath to prepare for the next
Sun Salutation. This is like the first,
but your opposite leg leads. Once you
have mastered the sequence, try to
tune the moves to your breathing.

LEGS •
Keep your knees
straight and your
feet together.

FEET •
Keep your feet
together.

GREETING THE SUN

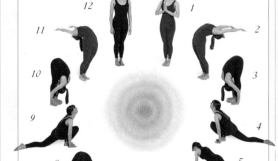

Attempt to do at least
6 Sun Salutations at
the beginning of every
yoga session. The ideal
number to perform is
12. Traditionally, the
sequence is practiced
in the morning, while
facing the rising sun.
As well as preparing you
for the ensuing **asanas**,
the sequence creates a
feeling of harmony with
nature. Move smoothly
and gracefully. Make
sure that you do not do
any variations of the
poses, as this will break
the momentum.

3

LEG RAISES

Definition: *Leg lifts performed lying on your back*

IN ORDER TO ENSURE THAT you obtain the maximum benefit from **asanas**, your body needs to become stronger as well as more flexible. The Sun Salutation has provided you with initial limbering up; practicing the leg raises will develop your physical strength and make it easier for you to perform asanas correctly. These exercises are especially good for strengthening your abdominal and **lumbar** muscles. It is important to keep your back as flat as possible on the floor, and your shoulders and neck relaxed. If you are unable to lift your legs all the way up while keeping your back flat on the ground, raise your legs only as high as you can manage.

OBJECTIVE: To strengthen your abdominal and **lumbar** muscles. *Rating* •

SINGLE LEG RAISES

Lie on your back and put your feet together. Push your back into the ground to keep your spine straight, then inhale as you lift one leg as high as possible. Try to synchronize your movements with your breathing. To finish, exhale as you lower your leg.

• BACK
Keep your back pushed into the ground.

• STRAIGHT
Keep your foot straight as you raise your leg.

• HANDS
Lay your hands next to your body with the palms down.

EACH LEG
Begin by raising your legs individually. Lift each leg at least 3 times.

LEG STRETCHING

Inhale, raising one leg. Grasp it, and
stretch it toward your head. Lift your
head to your leg. Hold for 10 seconds.
Exhale as you lower your
head and your leg.

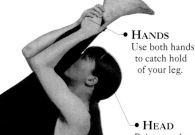

HANDS
Use both hands
to catch hold
of your leg.

HEAD
Raise your head
as you grasp
your leg.

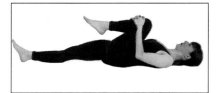

WIND RELIEVING

Hug one knee to your chest, and raise
your head up to your knee. Hold the
pose for about 10 seconds. Exhale as
you release your
leg, straighten
it, and lower
it. Repeat
the pose with
your other leg.

STARTING POSE
As you inhale, bend one
knee up to your chest, and
hold it with both hands.

KNEE
Your knee is
as close to your
chest as possible.

LOWER LEG •
Keep your lower leg
close to the ground.

DOUBLE LEG RAISE

Lie with your feet together and your
hands flat on the floor next to your
body. Push your back down, breathe
in, and raise both legs. Exhale as you
lower your legs. Start with 5 raises,
and build up to 10. If you cannot
manage this exercise with your back
flat, just do the single leg raises until
your back becomes stronger.

BACK •
Ensure that your
back does not
arch upward.

NECK
Push the base
of your neck
into the floor.

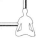

SKILL

4 THE HEADSTAND

Definition: *An asana in which you balance on your elbows, arms, and head*

KNOWN AS THE "KING OF **ASANAS**" because of its many benefits, the Headstand is the first of the 12 basic asanas and is considered by many to be a panacea for countless human ills. Sitting and standing for most of the day causes your circulation to become sluggish, so your heart has to work harder to pump sufficient blood to the upper parts of your body. Normally, your heart works against gravity; inverting your entire body lessens the strain on your heart, and allows a plentiful supply of oxygen-rich blood to reach your head and brain. This pose is not an advanced asana; even so, to begin with you may just wish to undertake the **Child's Pose** and the Dolphin, progressing to the full Headstand later.

OBJECTIVE: To relax and invigorate your entire body. *Rating* ••••

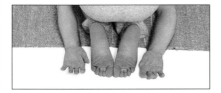

THE CHILD'S POSE

This is another relaxation pose, and is practiced before the Headstand and some other **asanas**. Sit on your heels, then bring your forehead forward to rest on the ground. While in this pose, relax in order to prepare yourself mentally for the Headstand.

HANDS
Lay your hands on the floor beside your feet, with the palms upward.

BUTTOCKS •
Bend forward from your hips, but make sure that your buttocks stay resting comfortably on your heels.

FOREHEAD •
Let your forehead touch the ground.

PROTECTION •
For comfort, you can use a rug or a mat during the Headstand.

THE DOLPHIN

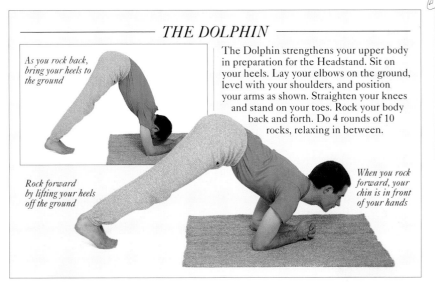

As you rock back, bring your heels to the ground

The Dolphin strengthens your upper body in preparation for the Headstand. Sit on your heels. Lay your elbows on the ground, level with your shoulders, and position your arms as shown. Straighten your knees and stand on your toes. Rock your body back and forth. Do 4 rounds of 10 rocks, relaxing in between.

Rock forward by lifting your heels off the ground

When you rock forward, your chin is in front of your hands

Step 1
ARMS & HANDS

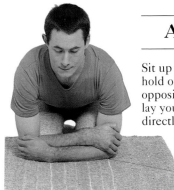

Sit up on your heels, then catch hold of both your elbows with the opposite hands. Lean forward and lay your forearms on the ground, directly beneath your shoulders. Let go of your elbows, and clasp your hands together.

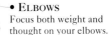

TRIPOD
Interlock your fingers to form a cap for your head to rest against.

• ELBOWS
Focus both weight and thought on your elbows.

Step 2
HEAD DOWN

HEAD REST
Rest your head in your hands.

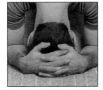

With your arms in the tripod position, above right, lower your head so that the top of your skull touches the ground and the back of it is cradled in your hands. Do not make any abrupt movements. Take the next steps slowly.

• WEIGHT
Little of your weight is on your head.

Step 3
ON YOUR TOES

From the crouched position with your head resting in your hands, straighten your knees and push your hips up above your head. Then, keeping your legs straight, stretch up high on your toes.

HIPS •
Keep your back straight and your hips directly over your head.

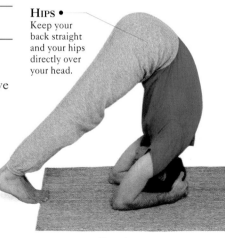

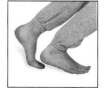

WALK IN
Walk your toes in toward your head. Do not drop your hips or bend your knees.

Step 4
HALF HEADSTAND

Now bend your knees, bringing them to your chest. Arch your back slightly, as you do when standing up; this will enable you to balance your body in this position. Do not proceed unless you can hold this position for at least 30 seconds without feeling any discomfort.

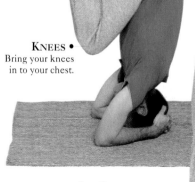

KNEES •
Bring your knees in to your chest.

• HEELS
Your heels remain tucked in close to your buttocks.

Step 5
KNEES UP

With your knees still bent, start to straighten your hips. Slowly and carefully, raise your knees until they are pointing straight up toward the ceiling.

• ARCH
Do not arch your back too much. It should keep the natural curve that it has when you stand upright.

ELBOWS •
Rest your weight on your elbows.

FEET •
Stretch your feet up, keeping them flat and parallel to the ceiling.

KNEES •
Keep your knees straight, and do not allow your legs to drop back.

HIPS •
Hold your hips straight above your head.

MUSCLES •
Tighten your abdominal muscles. This maintains correct posture, and prevents your back from arching too much.

Step 6

ALL THE WAY

Straighten your knees and lift your feet up toward the ceiling. Support your weight by bracing your elbows against the ground. At first, hold the Headstand for 30 seconds; as you become more skilled at adopting this pose, gradually increase the time to 3 minutes. Always come down before you start to feel tired. Leave the pose slowly and under control (see box).

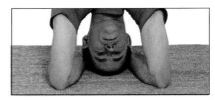

HEAD IN HANDS
Rest the back of your head against your hands. Relax, breathing through your nose.

• WEIGHT
Throughout the **asana**, keep most of your weight on your forearms and elbows, rather than on your head.

COMING OUT

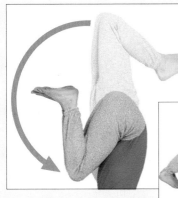

You should leave this **asana** as carefully as you entered it. Do not move jerkily or quickly, or you may lose control and fall.
• Bend your knees and lower them.
• Straighten your legs. Bring your feet to the ground, and then lower your knees.
• Lower your body so that your buttocks rest on your heels as in the **Child's Pose**.

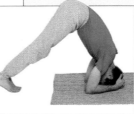

• Finally, relax your hands and return to the full Child's Pose.
• Do not lift your head up straight away. Rest for at least a minute.
• Relax in the **Corpse** before continuing.

Legs down (above). Feet to floor (right)

5 THE SHOULDER CYCLE

DAY 1

Definition: *Postures in which you balance on your shoulders*

SARVANGASAN, THE **SANSKRIT** NAME FOR the Shoulderstand, comes from the word "sarva", meaning whole. This **asana** strengthens your entire body; it gives many of the benefits of the Headstand, but here the circulation is directed to your thyroid gland instead of your brain. The Plough follows on from the Shoulderstand, and gives similar benefits. The cycle ends with the Bridge, which counters the two previous poses. All three improve the flexibility of your spine.

OBJECTIVE: To stretch your **cervical** and **thoracic** regions. *Rating* •••

THE SHOULDERSTAND

An inverted pose, with your body resting on your shoulders. Rating •

——— Step 1 ———
LEGS IN THE AIR

Before beginning the Shoulderstand, make sure that there is enough room behind you. You must be able to stretch your arms out behind your head and have at least 1ft (30cm) between your fingertips and any obstructions. Lie flat on your back, with your feet together. Inhale while bringing your legs up to a right angle.

• **LEGS**
Bring both legs up at a right angle to the ground.

• **BREATHING**
Breathe in as you raise your legs.

HANDS •
Lay your hands flat on the floor next to your sides.

• **BACK**
Keep your back flat on the floor.

Step 2
MOVING UP

Tuck your hands under your buttocks, with your fingers pointing toward your spine. Then, as you exhale, gently raise your body by letting your hands walk down your back and push you into position.

LEGS •
Your legs are straight but relaxed.

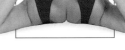

HANDS •
Your hands form a support for your back.

ELBOWS •
Your elbows are bent and flat on the floor.

Step 3
IN BALANCE

FEET •
Keep your feet close together.

Continue to move your hands up your back until you rest on your shoulders. Breathe normally, and keep your legs straight. Hold for 30 seconds; as the pose becomes easier, increase the time to 3 minutes. To come down, drop your feet halfway to the floor behind your head. Put your hands on the floor. Unroll your body **vertebra** by vertebra to the floor.

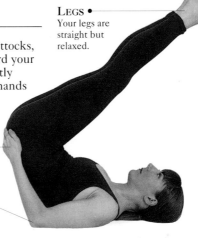

HAND POSITION
Put your hands on the small of your back, with your fingers toward your spine.

• HANDS
Support your body weight evenly with both your palms.

VARIATION
Inhale with your hands on your back. Exhale and bring one foot to the floor behind your head. Inhale. Raise your leg. Swap sides.

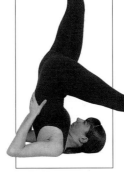

NECK •
Feel your body lift from the base of your neck. Press your chin into your neck.

THE PLOUGH

On your shoulders with your feet behind your head. Rating ••

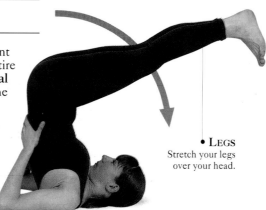

— Step 1 —
LEGS OVER

In the Plough, your body is bent forward; this stretches your entire spine, particularly your **cervical vertebrae** and shoulders. Come up into a Shoulderstand, and inhale deeply. Exhale while lowering your feet to the floor behind your head.

• LEGS
Stretch your legs over your head.

UPPER BACK •
The Plough helps to make your upper back more flexible, nourishing your spinal nerves.

HANDS
Lay your hands flat on the floor, palms downward.

— Step 2 —
LEGS DOWN

Rest your toes on the floor, then lay your arms down flat. Hold for 30 seconds at first, but aim to build up to 2 minutes. If you cannot lower your feet all the way, keep your hands on your back for support. To come out, lift your feet off the floor, and slowly roll down. Relax in the **Corpse**.

HEELS •
Push your heels back, as if trying to bring them to the ground.

PLOUGH VARIATION

You may try this variation if you are supple enough. Once in the Plough, lower your knees to the floor by your ears. Hook your arms over your legs. To come out, straighten your knees, then roll down as described above.

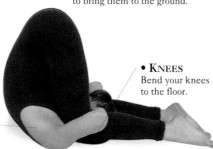

• KNEES
Bend your knees to the floor.

ARMS •
Hook your arms over your knees.

THE BRIDGE

Arching up with your head, shoulders, and feet on the ground. Rating •••

Step 1
ON YOUR BACK

Done straight after the Plough, the Bridge is a complementary stretch for your **thoracic** and **lumbar** regions, releasing any muscle tension that has built up. From the **Corpse Pose**, bend your knees and lay your feet on the floor by your buttocks.

STARTING POSE
Relax in the **Corpse Pose** before you attempt the Bridge.

FEET •
Your feet are positioned close to your buttocks.

Step 2
ARCH UP

Place your hands flat on your back, with your fingers pointing in toward your spine, as for the Shoulderstand. Keeping your head, shoulders, and feet on the floor, arch your hips and chest up as high as possible. Hold the position for 30 seconds.

• **FEET**
Keep your feet flat on the floor.

• **FINGERS AND THUMBS**
Your fingers point toward your spine, and your thumbs toward the ceiling.

BRIDGE VARIATION

Once you are supple enough, try this variation. Come into the Bridge, inhale, and raise one leg, keeping it straight. Exhale as you lower it. Repeat the pose with both legs, holding each leg in the air for a few seconds before lowering it.

• **LEGS**
Lift your leg up above your head, keeping it straight.

FOOT •
One foot stays flat on the floor to help support your weight.

THE FULL SEQUENCE

Putting together all three poses. Rating •••

COMBINING THE POSES

Once you have mastered the Shoulderstand, Plough, and Bridge, and feel comfortable in each position, all three **asanas** can be linked to form an uninterrupted sequence. The full series of poses is shown here.

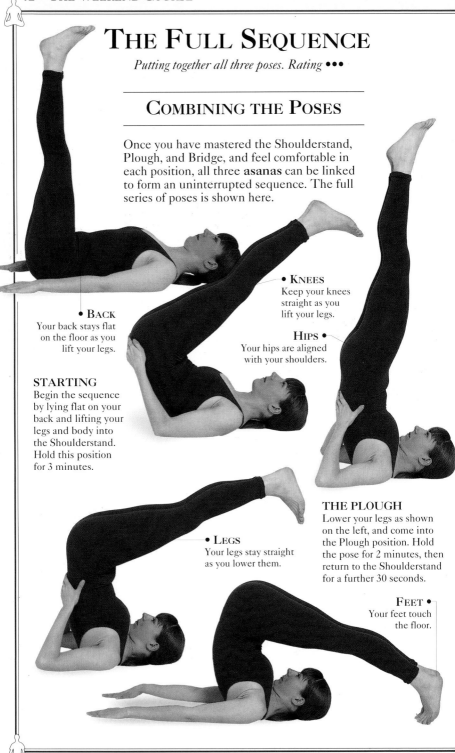

• KNEES
Keep your knees straight as you lift your legs.

HIPS •
Your hips are aligned with your shoulders.

• BACK
Your back stays flat on the floor as you lift your legs.

STARTING
Begin the sequence by lying flat on your back and lifting your legs and body into the Shoulderstand. Hold this position for 3 minutes.

THE PLOUGH
Lower your legs as shown on the left, and come into the Plough position. Hold the pose for 2 minutes, then return to the Shoulderstand for a further 30 seconds.

• LEGS
Your legs stay straight as you lower them.

FEET •
Your feet touch the floor.

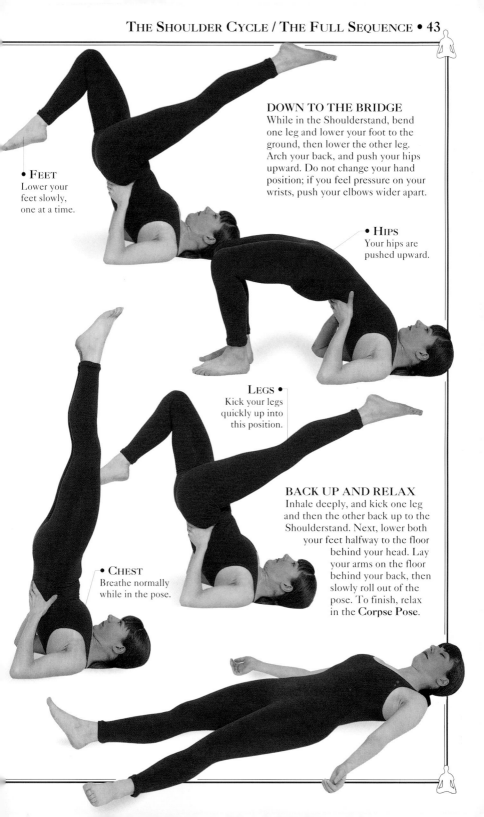

• FEET
Lower your
feet slowly,
one at a time.

DOWN TO THE BRIDGE
While in the Shoulderstand, bend
one leg and lower your foot to the
ground, then lower the other leg.
Arch your back, and push your hips
upward. Do not change your hand
position; if you feel pressure on your
wrists, push your elbows wider apart.

• HIPS
Your hips are
pushed upward.

LEGS •
Kick your legs
quickly up into
this position.

BACK UP AND RELAX
Inhale deeply, and kick one leg
and then the other back up to the
Shoulderstand. Next, lower both
your feet halfway to the floor
behind your head. Lay
your arms on the floor
behind your back, then
slowly roll out of the
pose. To finish, relax
in the **Corpse Pose**.

• CHEST
Breathe normally
while in the pose.

6

THE FISH

Definition: *Lying on your back and arching your chest*

THE FISH IS THE STRETCH that counters the Shoulderstand and Plough, and so follows them in a yoga session. The name of the posture derives from the fact that if you adopt the position in water, you will float quite easily. The **asana** does wonders for your respiratory system; when you assume this position, your chest is stretched open and your bronchial tubes are widened to promote easier breathing. In time your ribcage will expand, and this will also encourage you to breathe more deeply. By lifting your chest and tucking your arms underneath your body, you will combat postural defects such as rounded shoulders. In addition, the Fish removes stiffness from your shoulders and the **cervical** region of your spine, thus releasing pressure on your nerves. Try to hold the pose for half of the time that you spent in the Shoulderstand, in order to equalize the stretching effects on your spine and muscles.

OBJECTIVE: To ease tension and improve spinal flexibility. *Rating* •

— Step 1 —

ON YOUR BACK

Assume the **Corpse Pose** and, when you are ready, begin to come into the Fish. Stay flat on your back, and bring your feet together. With your arms straight by your sides, lay your palms on the floor, then tuck your hands in underneath your buttocks.

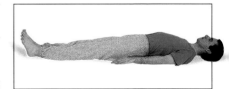

STARTING POSE
Prepare yourself for this **asana** by relaxing in the **Corpse Pose** for as long as you need.

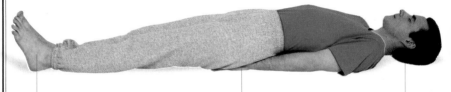

• **FEET**
Lie with your feet together and toes pointing upward.

HANDS •
Keeping your arms straight, put your hands under your buttocks.

HEAD •
Begin with your head upward.

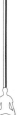

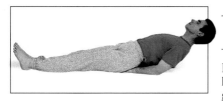

CHEST LIFT
Press your elbows down on the floor, inhale, and arch your chest upward as far as you can.

HEAD BACK

Having arched your spine, tilt your head so that your crown rests on the ground. Hold for 30 seconds. To come out of the Fish, slide your head back and then lower your chest. To finish, relax by lying in the **Corpse**.

LEGS •
Your legs are straight but stay relaxed.

FISH VARIATION

Try this variation if you are flexible enough. In the **Easy Pose**, clasp your toes. Lie back, arch up, and rest your buttocks on your heels. Lay the top of your head on the floor.

HANDS •
Your hands hold on to your toes.

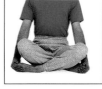

• CHEST
Your chest arches up as much as possible.

KNEES BENT
Sit cross-legged, then put your arms down behind your knees and catch hold of your toes.

FISH IN LOTUS

This pose is an advanced variation on the ordinary Fish. It is similar to the **Easy Pose** variation shown above, except that it begins with the Lotus (see p.49). Practitioners of yoga use this variation for staying afloat in water. The Fish in Lotus pose should not be attempted by beginners, or even by more experienced yoga students, until the full Lotus position can be held comfortably for a long period of time.

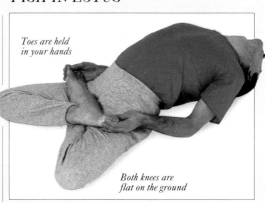

Toes are held in your hands

Both knees are flat on the ground

SKILL

7

BEND & STRAIGHTEN

DAY 1

Definition: *Stretching your spine forward*

THE FORWARD BEND LOOKS, AND IS, SIMPLE – provided you relax into the position, rather than forcing yourself into it. The pose is one of the most powerful and important **asanas**, helping to ease the spinal compression caused by standing upright. Its practice contributes greatly toward keeping your back supple, your joints mobile, your nervous system invigorated, and your internal organs toned. The Inclined Plane is the counterpose to the Forward Bend. It complements the forward stretch that your body is given in the previous pose, and increases the strength and flexibility of your arms. In this **asana** your hips are pushed upward, and your body is held straight and balanced on your hands and feet.

OBJECTIVE: To stretch the back of your body. *Rating* •

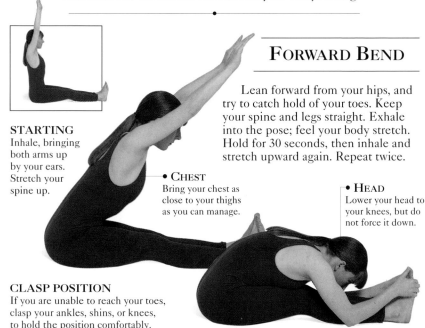

FORWARD BEND

STARTING
Inhale, bringing both arms up by your ears. Stretch your spine up.

Lean forward from your hips, and try to catch hold of your toes. Keep your spine and legs straight. Exhale into the pose; feel your body stretch. Hold for 30 seconds, then inhale and stretch upward again. Repeat twice.

• **CHEST**
Bring your chest as close to your thighs as you can manage.

• **HEAD**
Lower your head to your knees, but do not force it down.

CLASP POSITION
If you are unable to reach your toes, clasp your ankles, shins, or knees, to hold the position comfortably.

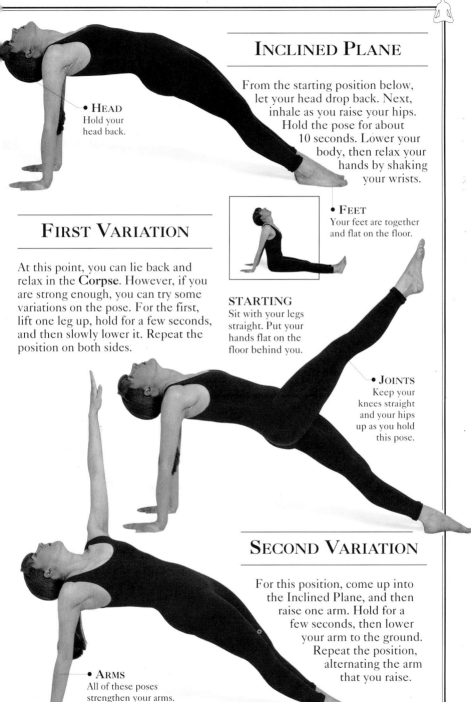

INCLINED PLANE

From the starting position below, let your head drop back. Next, inhale as you raise your hips. Hold the pose for about 10 seconds. Lower your body, then relax your hands by shaking your wrists.

- **HEAD**
Hold your head back.

FIRST VARIATION

At this point, you can lie back and relax in the **Corpse**. However, if you are strong enough, you can try some variations on the pose. For the first, lift one leg up, hold for a few seconds, and then slowly lower it. Repeat the position on both sides.

- **FEET**
Your feet are together and flat on the floor.

STARTING
Sit with your legs straight. Put your hands flat on the floor behind you.

- **JOINTS**
Keep your knees straight and your hips up as you hold this pose.

SECOND VARIATION

For this position, come up into the Inclined Plane, and then raise one arm. Hold for a few seconds, then lower your arm to the ground. Repeat the position, alternating the arm that you raise.

- **ARMS**
All of these poses strengthen your arms.

SKILL

8 SITTING POSES

DAY 1

Definition: *Exercises performed while seated*

MANY PEOPLE TODAY spend a lot of time sitting hunched in chairs. This shortens and weakens their back muscles. The seated poses featured here can help to remedy poor posture brought on by such inactivity. This lesson closes the first day; remember to finish by relaxing in the **Corpse Pose**, as you should after every yoga session.

OBJECTIVE: To stretch your back muscles. *Rating* ••••

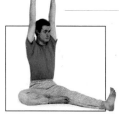

ONE KNEE BENT

Assume the starting pose, and stretch your spine up as far as you can. Then exhale while bending forward over your straight leg, and grasp your toes. Hold for 30 seconds. Inhale as you come up. Repeat with the other leg.

STARTING POSE
Sit with straight legs. Put one foot against your other thigh, then inhale as you lift your arms straight up.

• **SPINE**
Keep your spine as straight as you can manage.

CHEST •
Bring your chest down to lie on your leg.

FEET APART

Sit with your legs wide apart. Inhale as you lift your arms over your head, then exhale as you stretch forward. Grasp your toes, and lower your head toward the ground.

• **NECK**
Relax your neck, letting your head hang down.

FEET •
Catch hold of your feet with your hands.

THE BUTTERFLY

Sit up straight, bend both knees, and bring the soles of your feet together. Next, catch hold of your feet with both hands and draw them in close to your body, then gently bounce your knees down toward the ground. Make sure that your hands are holding your feet firmly, and that your feet are as close to your body as possible.

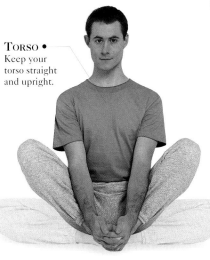

TORSO •
Keep your torso straight and upright.

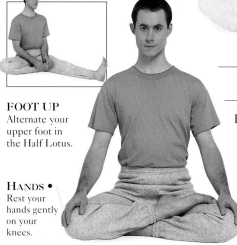

FOOT UP
Alternate your upper foot in the Half Lotus.

HANDS •
Rest your hands gently on your knees.

THE HALF LOTUS

Bring one foot up to rest on the opposite thigh. Tuck your other foot under your upper thigh. This pose is known as the Half Lotus. If you are supple enough, you can use it instead of the **Easy Pose** during your breathing and warming up exercises.

THE LOTUS POSE

The Full Lotus is an advanced position, which should not be attempted until you have been practicing yoga for some time, and have mastered all of the other seated poses shown here. This classic pose involves resting the backs of both feet high up on their opposite thighs.
The lotus flower is a significant symbol in the culture and mythology of India. The plant has its roots in mud, but the flower constantly strives to lift its head toward the light of the sun. Unaffected by the mire from which it rises, the lotus is considered beautiful because of this struggle. In yoga it represents self-awareness, and its namesake is adopted for **meditation** and breathing exercises.

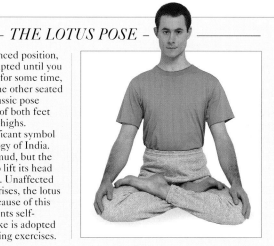

SKILL

9 STRETCHING BACK

Definition: *Asanas to stretch your spine backward*

THE COBRA AND LOCUST are the first two new poses for day two. Before attempting them, remember to do the breathing exercises, preparation for the session, and the Sun Salutation, followed by the poses covered on day one. The Cobra is a face-down position in which you lift your upper body. The pose works both the deep and the superficial muscles of your back, toning and strengthening the abdomen. In the Locust you lift your lower body, working your back muscles and stimulating your internal organs.

OBJECTIVE: To increase flexibility in your spinal column. *Rating* •••

THE COBRA

Coiling your upper body up and back. Rating •••

———— Step 1 ————
FACE DOWN

Lie on your front in the **Corpse Pose** for at least 2 minutes. Then, when you are fully relaxed, begin to come into the Cobra. Still lying on your front, place your hands flat on the floor so that they are directly underneath your shoulders. Next, lift your head up a little and bend your neck, then lower your forehead to the ground.

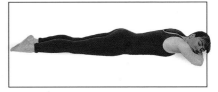

STARTING POSE
Relax in the frontal **Corpse Pose** (see p.54). Lie on your abdomen, then place one hand on top of the other to make a pillow. Turn your head and rest your cheek on your hands.

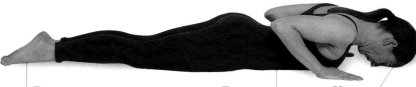

• FEET
Place your feet with toes together and heels apart.

ELBOWS •
Tuck your elbows in close to your body.

HEAD •
Rest your forehead on the ground.

Step 2
ROLL UP

Inhale, slowly rolling up and back. First, bring your forehead up, so that your nose rests on the floor. Next, raise your nose, then continue to roll up and back. Move slowly, so that you feel each **vertebra** arching back.

• ABDOMEN
Your abdomen remains in contact with the ground throughout this pose.

• SHOULDERS
Ensure that you do not hunch your shoulders.

LEGS •
Your legs stay straight and flat on the ground.

BACK •
Your back is arched, and your chest stretches out.

HOLD
Hold the pose for 10 seconds. Slowly roll down, keeping your head back until last. Repeat 3 times.

GOING FURTHER

Once you are proficient in the above steps, you can attempt some variations.
• In the Cobra, turn your head to look over your right shoulder, trying to see your left heel. Hold for about 10 seconds, then return your head to the center and repeat while looking over the other shoulder.
• From the starting position, lift your hands off the ground and roll your body up using only your back muscles.
• Always return to a resting position on your abdomen after these poses.
• With practice you may be able to attempt the variation shown here, in which your feet touch your head.

SKILL
THE LOCUST

Lying face down with lifted legs. Rating ••••

Step 1
FACE DOWN

Lie on your front. Rest your chin on the ground, then move it forward as much as you can, so that your throat lies almost flat. Put your arms by your sides, then push your hands under your body, and make them into fists or clasp them together. Bring your elbows as close together as possible.

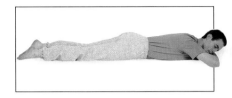

STARTING POSE
Begin in the frontal **Corpse** (see p.54).

HEAD •
Stretch your head forward.

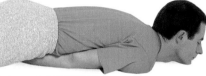

CLENCH
To help you lever your body upward, clench your fists together and push against the ground with your hands.

CLASP
You may find that clasping your hands together is more comfortable or that it allows better leverage.

Step 2
HALF LOCUST

Inhale as you lift one leg. Hold this position for at least 10 seconds, then exhale while lowering your leg and repeat the pose with your other leg. Practice it 3 times on each side.

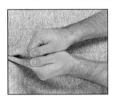

RAISED LEG •
Your raised leg is kept straight.

LOWER LEG •
Ensure that your lower leg remains flat on the floor.

HIPS •
Do not let your hips twist as you raise your leg.

CHIN
The further forward you push your chin, the more your spine can stretch and the more you will gain from this **asana**.

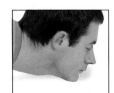

—— Step 3 ——
FULL LOCUST

Lie with your chin out, as in the Half
Locust, then take 3 deep breaths. On
the third, lift both legs off the ground.
They may not come up far at first, but
with practice you may be able to lift
them much higher. Hold for as long
as you can, then lower your feet.
Repeat twice and then relax.

• FEET
Place your
feet together.

KNEES •
Hold your knees
straight, and raise
your legs as high
as you can.

• CHIN
Rest your chin
on the ground.

ELBOWS •
Keep your elbows
close together.

UP AND UP
With practice, you will
be able to raise your
legs higher. Eventually,
you may even be able to
lift your body vertically.

THE ADVANCED LOCUST

This more difficult pose
must be attempted only
by experienced students
of yoga. The aim, in the
advanced **asana**, is to
raise your feet straight up
and then lower them over
your head. This backward
bend compresses your
vertebrae while stretching
the front of your body to
its greatest extent. The
strength and flexibility
necessary for this pose
will eventually develop
with regular practice.

*Push your hands
down against the
floor for leverage*

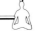

SKILL

10 BACK BENDS

Definition: *Backward bending poses*

TO KEEP YOUR BODY HEALTHY, your back must be strong and supple, with the ability to bend backward as well as forward. In other words, it should be balanced. The Bow works all parts of your back simultaneously. In this **asana**, your head, chest, and legs are lifted, while your body rests on your abdomen. The pose is so named because as you hold it, your body is bent back like a bow and your arms are held straight and taut like a bowstring. Initially, you may wish to attempt only the first three steps, moving on to the Rocking Bow when you have become more confident and lithe. The Wheel and its variations may appear difficult, but when worked on systematically they can bring both strength and flexibility to your spine and back muscles. All of these poses combine and augment the benefits gained from the Cobra and the Locust.

OBJECTIVE: To increase flexibility in your spine and hips. *Rating* ••••

FRONTAL CORPSE

Before and after all **asanas** you must relax for as long as necessary. The position that you adopt for relaxing between back bends is a variation on the **Corpse Pose**, in which you lie on your front. Like all Corpse variations, this pose prepares you mentally and physically for performing an asana.

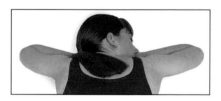

HEAD ON HANDS
Your hands make a pillow on which you can rest your head as you relax in this position.

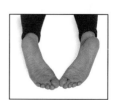

FEET
Position your feet with your big toes together; let your heels and ankles fall gently out to either side.

• **ABDOMEN**
Breathe deeply, focusing all your thoughts on your abdomen.

HEAD •
Lay your head down first on one side and then on the other.

THE BOW

Balancing on your abdomen, in the shape of a bow. Rating ●●●

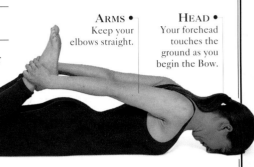

Step 1
CATCH HOLD

ARMS •
Keep your
elbows straight.

HEAD •
Your forehead
touches the
ground as you
begin the Bow.

To begin, lie on your front with your
forehead on the ground. Now bend
your knees and catch hold of your
ankles. Make sure that
you do grasp your ankles
rather than the top of
your feet or your toes.
Keep your feet relaxed.

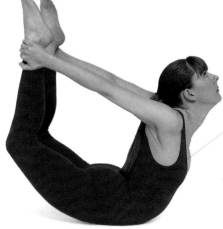

Step 2
LIFT UP

Inhale, raising your head, chest, and
legs. Straighten your knees. Hold for
10 seconds, aiming to increase to 30.
Breathe as you hold the pose. Exhale,
and lower your body. Repeat 3 times.

• CHEST
Lift your chest as
high as you can.

GRIP
Hold your ankles
firmly as you rock.

ROCKING BOW

For this exercise, come into the Bow,
arching as high as you can. Keep your
head back and gently rock, using your
breath to propel your body. Exhale as
you rock forward, and inhale as you
rock back. Do not forget to relax in
the **Corpse Pose** on your front after
you have completed this movement.

LEGS •
Lift your legs and hips
up as high from the
ground as possible.

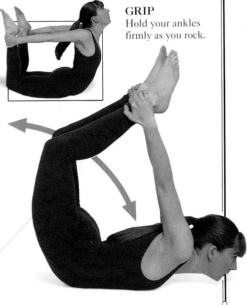

SKILL
10 WHEEL POSES
Auxiliary exercises to give your spine a full backward bend. Rating ••••

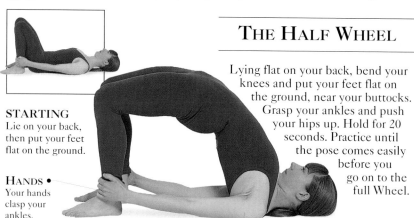

STARTING
Lie on your back,
then put your feet
flat on the ground.

HANDS •
Your hands
clasp your
ankles.

THE HALF WHEEL

Lying flat on your back, bend your
knees and put your feet flat on
the ground, near your buttocks.
Grasp your ankles and push
your hips up. Hold for 20
seconds. Practice until
the pose comes easily
before you
go on to the
full Wheel.

——— Step 1 ———
STARTING POSE

Lie on your back, then bend
your legs and put your feet by
your buttocks. Bend your
arms, and turn your hands so
that your fingers point toward
your shoulder blades. Lay
your hands flat on the floor
behind your shoulders.

• SHOULDERS
Your shoulders must stay on
the ground during this pose.

HANDS •
Your hands lie flat on the
ground, with your fingers
pointing at your feet.

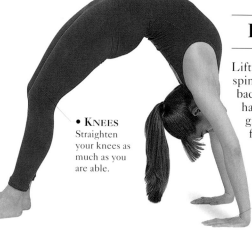

• KNEES
Straighten
your knees as
much as you
are able.

——— Step 2 ———
INTO THE WHEEL

Lift your hips, arching your entire
spine up and dropping your head
back. In the full Wheel, only your
hands and feet remain on the
ground. Aim to hold the pose
for 30 seconds. Your hands
and feet will be parallel.

• HANDS
Walk your hands in
toward your feet.

Step 1
KNEEL & LEAN

To assume the Camel, a pose also known as the Kneeling Wheel, start by sitting on your heels. Place both hands behind your body and, resting on them, drop your head back. Raise your hips, arching them forward.

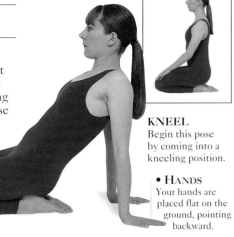

KNEEL
Begin this pose by coming into a kneeling position.

• HANDS
Your hands are placed flat on the ground, pointing backward.

HIPS •
Begin with your hips and buttocks resting on your heels.

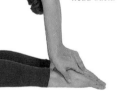

• HEAD
Lean your head back.

Step 2
INTO THE CAMEL

Walk your hands in toward your feet, and try to catch hold of your heels. At the same time, push your hips up and forward as far as possible, and allow your head to drop back. If this pose is done correctly, your body will take on a shape resembling a rectangle.

• HANDS AND HEELS
Move your hands toward your feet until you are able to take hold of your heels.

THE DIAMOND

The advanced variation on the Wheel is known as the Diamond, and must only be attempted when you are able to hold the Wheel easily. In this pose your body forms the shape of a diamond, hence the name. The aim is to bend your spine backward until your head touches the floor, then grasp your feet with your hands. The pose is completed by pulling with your hands so that your head comes down to rest on top of your heels.

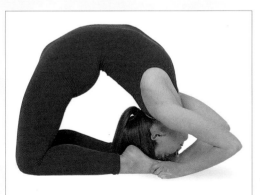

11 JOINT MOBILITY

Definition: *Stretches for your shoulders and hips*

IT IS SAID THAT PEOPLE in the modern world carry the majority of their tension in their shoulders. This stress leads to problems such as hunched shoulders and stiff necks, which result in pain and excessive strain on the body. The Cow's Head and its variations relieve stiffness in your chest, neck, and upper back region. Practicing these **asanas**, and their counterpose, the Frog, will open your chest and straighten rounded shoulders. The poses will also enhance mobility and flexibility in your leg muscles and joints.

OBJECTIVE: To bring flexibility to your joints. *Rating* ••••

THE COW'S HEAD

Sit up on your heels. Bring your right arm over your head, bending your elbow. Put your left arm behind your back and clasp your hands. In this position, bend forward. Hold for 30 seconds and then sit up on your heels, releasing your hands. Shake out your arms and repeat on the other side.

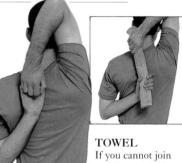

TOWEL
If you cannot join your hands, hold a rolled towel behind you, gripping one end with each hand.

HANDS •
Keep your hands clasped while you are in this pose.

BUTTOCKS •
Sit with your buttocks resting on your heels.

HEAD TO FLOOR
To complete this **asana**, try to bring your forehead down as close to the floor as you can manage.

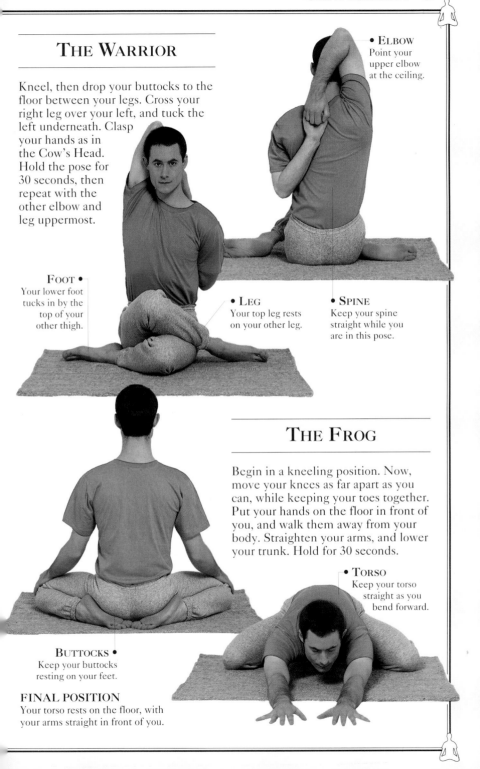

THE WARRIOR

Kneel, then drop your buttocks to the floor between your legs. Cross your right leg over your left, and tuck the left underneath. Clasp your hands as in the Cow's Head. Hold the pose for 30 seconds, then repeat with the other elbow and leg uppermost.

• **ELBOW**
Point your upper elbow at the ceiling.

FOOT •
Your lower foot tucks in by the top of your other thigh.

• **LEG**
Your top leg rests on your other leg.

• **SPINE**
Keep your spine straight while you are in this pose.

BUTTOCKS •
Keep your buttocks resting on your feet.

FINAL POSITION
Your torso rests on the floor, with your arms straight in front of you.

THE FROG

Begin in a kneeling position. Now, move your knees as far apart as you can, while keeping your toes together. Put your hands on the floor in front of you, and walk them away from your body. Straighten your arms, and lower your trunk. Hold for 30 seconds.

• **TORSO**
Keep your torso straight as you bend forward.

SKILL

12 SPINAL TWISTING

DAY 2

Definition: *A lateral stretch for your entire spine*

AFTER BENDING FORWARD AND BACK, your spine requires a lateral twist to retain its mobility. This ability to twist is often the first type of flexibility to be lost. During the Spinal Twists your **vertebrae** are mobilized; the exercises also allow more nourishment to reach the roots of the spinal nerves and the **sympathetic nervous system**.

OBJECTIVE: To maintain sideways mobility in your spine. *Rating* •

— Step 1 —

ONE LEG STRAIGHT

Relax in the **Child's Pose** before starting, then sit up with your legs straight in front of you. Bend your right knee, and put your right foot on the ground on the outside of your left knee.

• RIGHT LEG
Your right leg is bent and crosses over your left thigh.

• LEFT LEG
Your left leg is straight out in front of you.

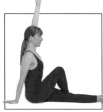

ARMS
Place your right hand flat behind you. Raise your left arm in the air.

BUTTOCKS •
Both buttocks stay on the ground.

— Step 2 —

TWIST ROUND

Twist to the right. Lower your left arm in front of your knee, and grip your right ankle. Look over your right shoulder. Hold for 30 seconds, then repeat on the left side.

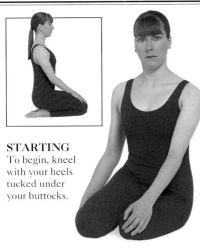

STARTING
To begin, kneel
with your heels
tucked under
your buttocks.

LEGS BENT

This type of spinal twist, in which
both your legs are bent, must not be
attempted until you can hold the
previous pose comfortably. Sit on
your heels. Drop your buttocks to
the floor to the left of your legs.

• HIPS
Move your hips so that your
buttocks rest by your legs.

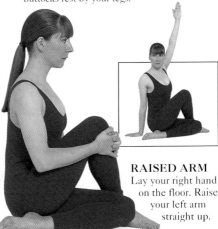

LEG POSITION

Bend your right leg. Cross your
right foot over your left leg, and
place it on the floor by the outside
of your left knee. Keeping your
arm straight, put your right hand
flat on the floor behind your back.

STRAIGHT BACK •
Keep your back straight
and upright.

RAISED ARM
Lay your right hand
on the floor. Raise
your left arm
straight up.

HEAD •
Look over
your right
shoulder.

THE TWIST

Lower your left arm, bringing it
outside your bent knee, then
grasp your right ankle. Hold for
at least 30 seconds. Repeat,
twisting the other way.

SHOULDERS •
Twist your
shoulders
as much as
possible.

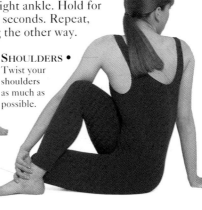

BUTTOCKS •
Both buttocks
stay resting on
the ground.

HAND •
Catch hold of your
ankle with your
opposite hand.

SKILL

13 BALANCING POSES

DAY 2

Definition: *Balancing your entire body on your hands*

ALL **ASANAS** SERVE TO IMPROVE physical and mental health, and increase your ability to focus the mind. Balancing exercises are particularly beneficial. Both of the poses shown here enhance concentration. The first pose, the Crow, develops mental tranquillity and also strengthens your wrists and forearms. The second, called the Peacock, demands a strong, flexible body and a disciplined mind. In this asana your elbows are bent into your abdomen. This allows a fresh supply of blood to the area, nourishing and toning your internal organs and eliminating sluggishness.

OBJECTIVE: To improve balance and concentration. *Rating* •••••

THE CROW

Balancing in a squatting position. Rating ••••

―――――― Step 1 ――――――
SQUAT TO START

To prepare yourself for the Crow, squat with your feet and knees wide apart. Position your arms between your knees, with your hands directly under your shoulders, then put your hands flat on the floor in front of you.

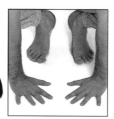

HANDS
Stretch your fingers wide and turn your hands inward slightly.

• KNEES
Bring your knees as far apart as you can comfortably manage.

FEET •
Lift your heels and rest your weight on the balls of your feet.

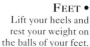

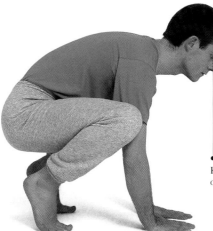

Step 2
KNEES TO ARMS

Bend your elbows, and turn them outward. Rest your knees against your upper arms. Next, rock forward until you feel your weight on your wrists. Stay in this position if you are unable to proceed further.

• EYES
Keep your eyes focused on a point in front of you.

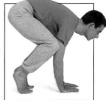

WEIGHT
This exercise is still useful even if you stop at this point, as your wrists support your weight and your forearm muscles are being stretched.

Step 3
RAISE YOUR FEET

Slowly raise each foot, then balance on your hands for at least 10 seconds. Aim to increase your time in the pose to 30 seconds; with practice you will be able to hold the position for up to a minute. To come out, lower your feet to the ground, sit up, and shake out your wrists. If you are strong enough, repeat the Crow twice.

HEAD •
Ensure that your head stays up. If it drops, you will be more likely to roll forward.

PROTECTION

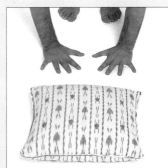

FEAR OF FALLING
If you are worried about falling onto your face, put a cushion in front of you.

• KNEES
Your knees rest against your upper arms.

• FEET
Your feet are held in midair, with your toes pointing down.

• HANDS
Your hands and wrists will support your weight.

13

THE PEACOCK

Balancing with your body parallel to the ground. Rating •••••

• **TORSO**
Sit up, keeping
your torso straight
and relaxed.

—————— Steps 1 & 2 ——————

HANDS TO THE FLOOR

Start in a kneeling position, then
move your knees apart. Place your
arms between your legs, bringing
your elbows and forearms together
and tucking your elbows in close
to your abdomen. Next, lay
your hands flat on the floor,
with your wrists together
and your fingers pointing
back toward your body.

• **FOREARMS**
Your forearms are
almost at right
angles to the floor.

STARTING POSE
Sit on your heels with
your knees wide apart.

—————— Steps 3 & 4 ——————

STRETCH OUT

Keep your hands directly under
your abdomen. Put your
forehead on the ground.
Next, stretch one leg and
then the other straight
out behind you. Your
weight should now be
resting on your hands,
toes, and forehead.

HEAD •
Your forehead
touches the floor.

LEGS •
Stretch your legs straight
behind you, supporting
them with your toes.

TOUCHING THE GROUND
At this point you are resting your weight
on your hands, toes, and forehead.

Steps 5 & 6

IN THE AIR

Raise your head, and shift your weight forward. Lift your toes. If you perform the movements slowly, you will raise your legs without effort. Hold for 10 seconds. With practice, you will be able to hold the pose for up to 30 seconds.

ARMS •
Your elbows are together and your weight is on your wrists.

EYES •
Focus on a point ahead to aid your concentration.

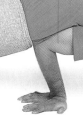

• LEGS
Your legs are held straight and parallel to the ground.

PARALLEL BODY
In the final position, your body is held straight and parallel to the floor.

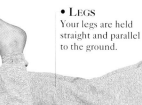

THE ADVANCED PEACOCK

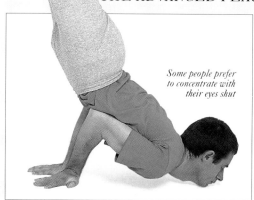

Some people prefer to concentrate with their eyes shut

With practice, you may be able to try this variation on the Peacock. The pose does, however, call for a great deal of strength and agility, and must only be attempted by advanced yoga students. Such people may even find this version of the Peacock easier than the ordinary **asana**, as the legs are in balance with the body rather than hanging behind it. In this pose, you balance on your hands and chin, with your legs raised vertically behind you.

SKILL

14

STANDING ASANAS

Definition: *Poses practiced in an upright position*

STANDING POSES DEVELOP strength and flexibility in your legs and hips, and equilibrium in your body. The Hands-to-Feet Pose stretches your spine and joints, and increases the blood supply to your brain. The Triangle is the last of the basic **asanas**. You must master this pose and its variations before trying the advanced asanas.

OBJECTIVE: To make your spine and legs supple and strong. *Rating* ••

HANDS-TO-FEET

Bending forward in a standing position. Rating •

FORWARD & DOWN

This is similar to the Forward Bend, but here gravity helps to stretch your body down. Stand with your feet together. Inhale, while lifting your arms straight above your head. Exhale as you bend forward and down. Breathe normally while you are in the pose. Hold for at least 30 seconds; as you gain experience, increase the time to several minutes.

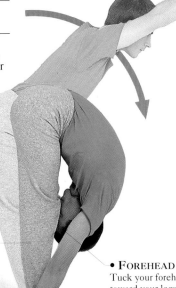

LEGS AND HIPS •
Keep your legs straight. Make sure that your hips are over your feet and do not move backward.

FEET •
Your weight is centered, and poised on the balls of your feet.

• **FOREHEAD**
Tuck your forehead in toward your legs as far as you can manage.

THE TRIANGLE

A lateral bend resembling a triangle. Rating ••

TO THE SIDE

The Triangle is a lateral stretch for your trunk muscles and spine, and makes your hips, legs, and shoulders more flexible. Stretch your right arm up, then bend to your left, sliding your left hand down your thigh. Do not twist your body. Hold for 30 seconds, working up to 2 minutes with practice. Inhale as you straighten up again. Repeat the pose on the other side.

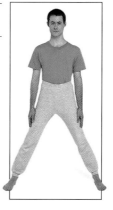

INITIAL POSE
Stand up straight, and place your feet slightly more than shoulder width apart.

ARM •
Raise your arm straight up above your head.

• HAND
Put your lower hand on your thigh to balance you as you bend.

BODY LINE
Your body forms a straight line, parallel to the floor, from your waist to your fingertips.

• HEAD
Keep your head in alignment with your straight spine.

KNEE •
Keep your knees straight while in this position.

• HAND
Your hand slides down toward your ankle.

SKILL
14 TRIANGLE VARIATIONS

Further poses to stretch and balance your body. Rating ••

STRETCH UP

Stand with your feet apart, turn your
left foot out, and bend your left knee.
Next, bend to the left and put
your left hand down by your
instep. Then lift your right
arm straight above your
head, and look up.
Hold for 30 seconds.
Repeat, bending
to the right.

ARM •
Your arm is held
straight out and
aligned with the
side of your chest.

• **HAND**
Keep your hand
flat on the floor.

• **EXTEND**
Stretch your straight leg
out as much as possible.

FINGERS •
Your fingers are closed and your
hand points up at the ceiling.

TWIST & LOOK UP

Stand with your feet apart. Hold
your arms straight out at shoulder
level, then twist to the left and
put your right hand down outside
your left foot. Keep your chest
and arms aligned, with your left
arm straight up and your
shoulders at 90° to the
floor. Hold the pose
for 30 seconds. Then
repeat it, but this time
twist to the right.

• **HEAD**
Turn your head
toward your
upper hand.

• **HAND**
Lay your hand flat on the floor,
on the outside of your foot.

TO THE SIDE

Stand with your feet apart, then turn your left foot out and bend your left knee. Next, twist to the left and put your right hand down outside or on your left foot. Raise your left arm straight up over your head. Repeat the pose, turning to both sides.

• **BODY**
Your body twists so that your right leg is aligned with your left arm.

• **FOOT**
Your foot is turned out as far as you find comfortable.

FOREHEAD •
Try to touch your knee or leg with your forehead.

HEAD-TO-KNEE

Stand with your feet apart and your hands clasped behind your back. Turn to one side, and exhale as you lower your forehead to your knee. Then lift your arms as far from your back as you can, and hold for 30 seconds. Inhale as you stand up. Repeat, turning to the other side.

A DEEP LUNGE

Stand with your feet wide apart and your left foot turned out. Clasp your hands behind your back. Next, bend from the hips and lower your head to the floor by that foot. Keep your right leg straight. Then lift your arms as high as you can, and hold for 30 seconds. Practice the pose on both sides.

ARMS •
Your arms are raised up and away from your back.

SKILL 14 THE STANDING POSES

During these exercises, you balance on one foot. Rating ••

BALANCING PRAYER

Stand on your left leg. Lift your arms over your head, and put your hands together. Keeping your body straight, lean forward and raise your right leg. Hold for 10 seconds, then swap legs.

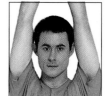

MIND POWER
Concentration is essential. Keep your balance by focusing your mind on a fixed point in front of you.

ARMS •
Hold your arms straight, beside your ears.

RAISED LEG •
Raise your right leg up behind you, keeping your knee straight.

• **FOOT**
Catch hold of your raised foot and lift it outward.

• **STRAIGHT LEG**
Keep your left leg straight and at 90° to the ground.

THE LORD NATARAJA

Stand on your left leg and bend your right knee. Bring your foot up to your buttock, and catch hold of it. Try to straighten your right knee, lifting your foot as far away from your body as you can. Then raise your left arm beside your left ear, and hold this position. In **Sanskrit**, "Nataraja" means "King of Dancers". This is another name for the god **Siva**, who, it is believed, first taught the yoga **asanas**.

BODY •
As your right leg rises, your trunk, right thigh, and raised left arm all stay aligned.

• **LEG**
Make sure that the leg on which you balance is straight.

THE TREE

Balancing on one foot, with arms lifted above your head. Rating ••

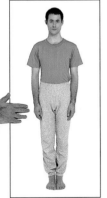

Step 1
FOOT TO THIGH

Balance on your left foot, and focus your mind on a fixed point. Bend your right knee, and put your foot on your left thigh. With practice, you will be able to put your foot at the top of your thigh in the Half Lotus position.

FOOT •
Hold your foot in place with both hands.

TO PREPARE
Stand straight. Focus your eyes on a point at eye level, such as a spot on a wall.

Step 2
HANDS OVER HEAD

Lift your arms up, and put your palms together. Hold the pose for a minute. If you wish, try the following exercise. Focus on a spot in front of you. In your mind, pull the spot in to rest between your eyebrows. Close your eyes, but keep your mind on this point.

• BREATHING
Breathe deeply while holding this pose to calm and focus your mind.

RAISED FOOT •
Keep the sole of your raised foot flat against your inner thigh.

• LEG
Balance on one foot, and keep your knee as straight as possible.

SKILL

15

DAY 2

FINAL RELAXATION

Definition: *Conscious relaxation while in the* **Corpse Pose**

KNOWING HOW TO RELAX is a vital part of keeping your body fit. Relaxation is primarily a mental process, as all muscle movements are controlled by your subconscious mind. By sending a message to each part of the body to relax, you can consciously ease any tension.

Do not omit this final skill – it is an essential element in your session, and will enhance all of the benefits gained from the **asanas**.

OBJECTIVE: To allow energy released by the **asanas** to flow free. *Rating* •

HEAD TO TOE

Lie in the **Corpse Pose**. Tense and relax all your muscles as shown, and do the head rolls. Then, in your mind, tell every part of your body to relax, starting with each toe. Feel the relaxation moving up your body. Finally, relax your jaw and let your mouth open slightly. Relax the back of your throat, then your tongue and face muscles. Stay in this pose for at least 10 minutes after each session.

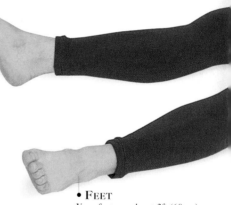

• FEET
Your feet are about 2ft (60cm) apart, with your toes turned out.

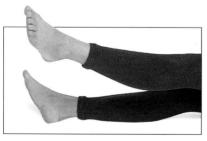

RAISE YOUR LEGS
Raise each leg 2in (5cm) from the ground, tense and release the muscles, and let it fall.

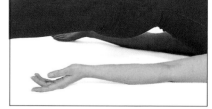

LIFT YOUR HIPS
Lift your buttocks, tense and relax them, and let them fall. Do the same with your chest.

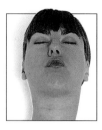

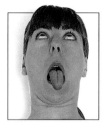

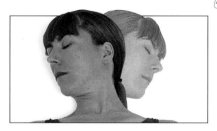

TENSE UP
Shut your eyes tight
and screw up all of
your face muscles.

STRETCH OUT
Open your eyes and
mouth wide. Stick
your tongue out fully.

ROLL YOUR HEAD
Slowly roll your head once or twice, touching
the ground with one ear and then the other,
then bring it to rest with your face upward.

• ARMS
Lay your arms at
45° to your body.

• BREATHING
Let your breathing
become slow and gentle.

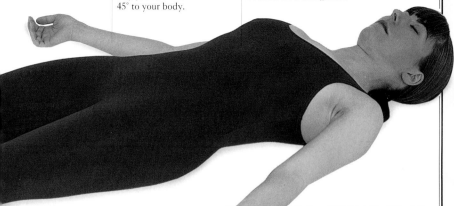

HANDS •
Your hands lie with
palms upward and
fingers curling gently.

—MIND & SLEEP—

• Slow breathing relaxes the mind.
Make your breathing very gentle and
quiet. Imagine that your mind is a
deep, still lake with no ripples. You
have no worries or fears. Soon you will
feel a sense of inner peace; enter into
that peace and become one with it.
• Once you have learned to relax, you
may find that you can put this skill to
use at other times as well. For instance,
if you have trouble falling asleep, lie
in bed and mentally go through the
steps of this guided relaxation.
• If you practice the **asanas** followed
by the relaxation period, you may find
that you need less sleep than before
and wake up feeling refreshed. This
is because these techniques help you
to go more quickly into deep sleep,
which is the most restful type of sleep.

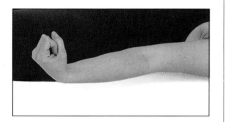

FOCUS ON HANDS
Lift each hand 2in (5cm). Make a fist, tense
your arm, then relax your hand and let it fall.

AFTER THE WEEKEND

What to do now you have finished your basic course

•

YOU HAVE NOW COMPLETED your introduction to the techniques of yoga **asanas** and **pranayama**. You will benefit most if you keep up your initial momentum with regular practice. If you feel stiff, do not be deterred; the best way to ease this is by doing a gentle asana session. Try to practice daily. Set aside a time when you will not be disturbed – perhaps first thing in the morning, or later in the evening before you have eaten. It is advisable to continue under the guidance of a qualified teacher, as he or she will be able to correct and improve your technique. The skills in this book are basic tools that can enhance your life, promoting good health and a positive attitude.

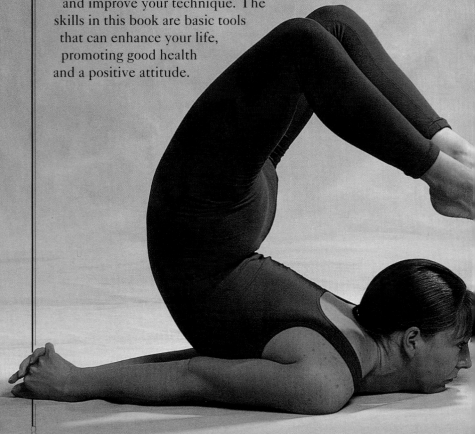

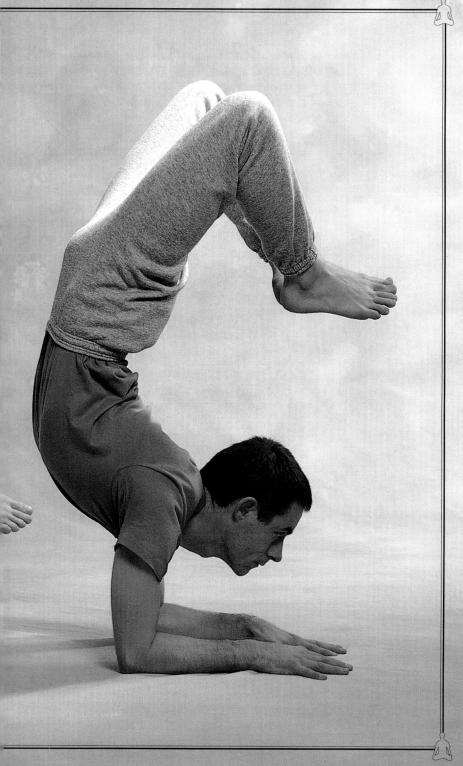

ORGANIZING YOUR PRACTICE

Fitting yoga sessions into your daily life

HERE ARE THREE suggested sessions, of different durations, for your yoga program. They include time allowed for **asanas** and time for relaxation between poses. Try the shorter routines when you are busy, but aim to do at least two full sessions per week for maximum benefit. Do not leave out the breathing exercises. If you are short of time, you can do them separately – for example, do the breathing in the morning and the asanas later on. If you have no time for any of the sessions, try to do at least six rounds of the Sun Salutation and a Headstand.

Breathing exercise

The Shoulderstand

	Fast	Average	Full
Relaxation	1 x 5 mins	1 x 5 mins	1 x 5 mins
Kapalabhati	3 x 1 min	3 x 1 min	3 x 1 min
Alternate nostril breathing	5 x ½ min	10 x ½ min	10 x ½ min
Preliminaries: neck & eyes	2 mins	5 mins	5 mins
The Sun Salutation	6 x ½ min	12 x ½ min	12 x ½ min
The Headstand	1 x 1 min	1 x 2 mins	1 x 3 mins
Leg raises	1½ mins	2 mins	2 mins
The Shoulderstand	1 x 1 min	1 x 2 mins	1 x 3 mins
The Plough	1 x ½ min	1 x ½ min	1 x 1 min
The Bridge	1 x ½ min	1 x ½ min	1 x ½ min
The Fish	1 x ½ min	1 x 1 min	1 x 1½ min
The Forward Bend	3 x 10 secs	3 x 20 secs	3 x ½ min

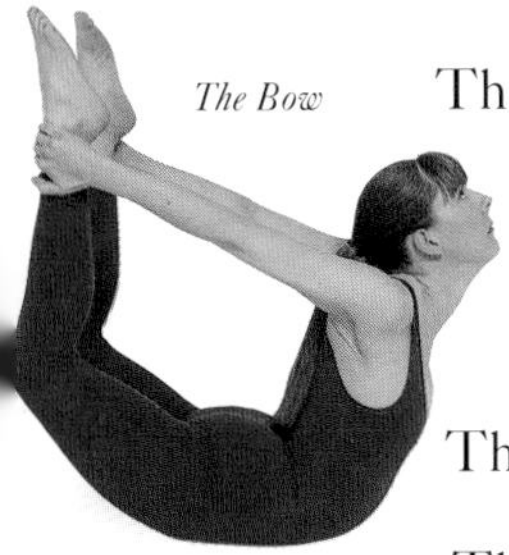

The Inclined Plane	1 x ½ min	1 x ½ min	1 x ½ min
Sitting poses		1 min	3 mins
The Cobra	2 x ½ min	3 x ½ min	3 x ½ min
The Half Locust		4 x 15 secs	4 x 15 secs
The Locust		2 x ½ min	2 x ½ min
The Bow		2 x ½ min	3 x ½ min
The Half Wheel			2 x ½ min
The Full Wheel			1 x 1 min
The Camel			3 x ½ min
The Cow's Head			2 x ½ min
The Frog			1 x 1 min
Spinal twisting	2 x ½ min	2 x ½ min	2 x 1 min
The Crow or Peacock		2 x ½ min	3 x ½ min
Hands-to-Feet	1 x ½ min	1 x 1 min	1 x 1 min
The Triangle	2 x ½ min	2 x ½ min	2 x ½ min
Triangle variations			2 x ½ min
The Tree			2 x 1 min
Standing asanas			3 x 1 min
Final relaxation	1 x 5 mins	1 x 10 mins	1 x 10 mins
Running Time	30 mins	53 mins	72 mins

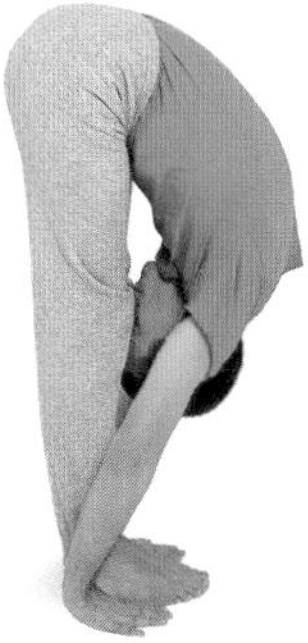

The Bow

Hands-to-Feet

Total session time allocated with relaxation between asanas	35 mins	60 mins	90 mins

ADVANCED ASANAS

Further yoga postures that you can achieve with practice

THERE ARE SAID TO BE 84,000 different yoga **asanas**. With this
many poses to choose from, you are unlikely ever to feel bored.
Once you have mastered the basic asanas covered in The Weekend
Course, you will be on the way to developing the flexibility,
strength, and confidence needed to attempt some of the
more advanced variations. The postures shown here are just
a few examples of what you can hope to achieve. Some
asanas may be possible after just a few months of lessons,
while perfecting others may take you years of tuition
and practice. Take your progress at your own
individual rate; remember that you must never
force yourself into difficult positions before
your body is ready. Never attempt any of
these poses unless you are receiving
guidance from a qualified teacher.

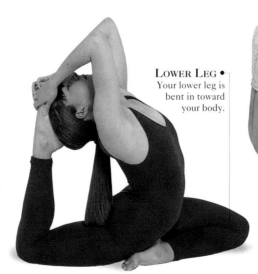

LOWER LEG •
Your lower leg is
bent in toward
your body.

• HIPS
Your hips arch
outward as your
entire body bends.

THE PIGEON
This **asana** is so named because your chest
is open and pushed forward like that of a
pigeon. Your hands, raised foot, and head all
come together in a powerful backward bend.

THE SCORPION
Once you can hold the Headstand
easily, you may be able to attempt the
Scorpion. This pose bends your spine
fully, and improves your circulation.

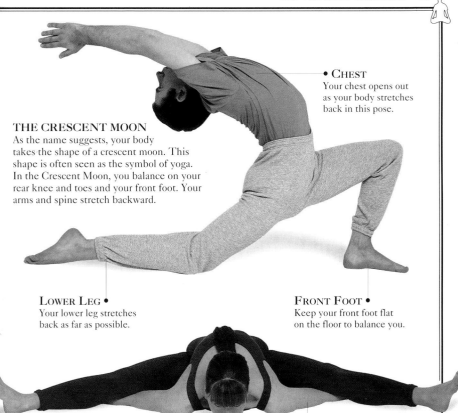

THE CRESCENT MOON

As the name suggests, your body takes the shape of a crescent moon. This shape is often seen as the symbol of yoga. In the Crescent Moon, you balance on your rear knee and toes and your front foot. Your arms and spine stretch backward.

• CHEST
Your chest opens out as your body stretches back in this pose.

LOWER LEG •
Your lower leg stretches back as far as possible.

FRONT FOOT •
Keep your front foot flat on the floor to balance you.

THE TORTOISE

Your legs are wide apart and your body bends down toward the floor. Your arms are tucked under your legs. With practice, it is possible to lay your chin and chest on the floor.

• ARMS
Your arms are tucked underneath your thighs in this forward bend.

THE PEACOCK IN LOTUS

In this variation on the Peacock, you balance your body on your hands as in the basic pose. This time, though, you start by crossing your legs in the Lotus position before you lift them off the ground.

FEET •
Your feet are tucked up and rest on the opposite thighs.

HANDS •
Your fingers are spread out to take your weight.

GOOD FOOD

Planning a balanced and nutritious diet for your body and mind

WHATEVER FORM OF PHYSICAL EXERCISE you practice, a healthy diet will increase your energy. Plan your diet so that it includes all the essential minerals and vitamins, as well as plenty of carbohydrates, protein, and fiber. Keep your intake of fat down by trying to avoid meat, fried foods, and snacks such as chocolate and crisps. Instead, eat plenty of fresh vegetables and fruit, and foods such as grains, nuts, and seeds.

• VEGETABLES
Providing vitamins, minerals, and fiber, vegetables are both delicious and vital for a healthy diet. Eat them raw or lightly cooked to retain their natural goodness.

CARBOHYDRATES •
Great energy-givers, pasta and rice can be satisfying elements in your diet. Other carbohydrates that you can include are bread and potatoes.

A YOGA DIET

The ideal diet for yoga is essentially vegetarian. Yoga philosophy identifies three categories of food.
• **Sattvic**, or pure, foods are items such as fresh fruit, grains, and vegetables. These form the bulk of a yoga diet.
• **Tamasic** – rotten or stale – foods include alcohol, meat, and tobacco.
• **Rajasic**, or overstimulating, foods include hot spices, coffee, and tea.

JUICY FRUIT •
Sweet but healthy, fruit is an ideal snack. Most varieties are low in fat but still high in vitamins and minerals.

BREAD AND CHEESE •
Cheese and other dairy products contain calcium for strong teeth and bones. Brown bread provides fiber as well as carbohydrates.

NUTS AND SEEDS •
Nuts and seeds also contain protein. There are many kinds to choose from, and they make a convenient snack.

• PULSES
Pulses give concentrated protein. For vegetarians they are a useful, filling alternative to meat.

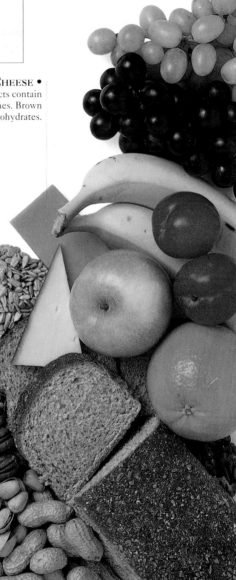
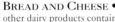

MEDITATION

Learning to focus and channel your mental energy

MEDITATION IS A STATE of consciousness; it allows you to go beyond the limits of normal awareness. Imagine that your mind resembles a lake. The bottom of the lake may be seen very clearly if the water is calm, but this will not be possible if the water is disturbed by waves. In the same way, when your mind is perfectly still you can bypass everyday distractions and perceive the source of true contentment. Meditation differs from deep sleep or relaxation in that it involves active mental effort rather than total rest. As well as relieving stress and replenishing energy, it can bring you physical, mental, and spiritual peace. To achieve inner serenity, you must learn to make your mind quiet and focus your mental energy inward. If you meditate for half an hour daily, your thinking will become clearer and you will be able to face life with greater spiritual strength.

AN IDEAL POSE

The ideal positions for meditation are the classic sitting postures, as these keep the **prana**, or vital energy, within your body. The Lotus, Half Lotus, and **Easy Pose** are all suitable. Place your hands in a comfortable position; some appropriate poses are shown here.

BREATHING •
Breathe quietly from your abdomen. Maintain a regular rhythm.

CHIN MUDRA
Form a circle with your thumb and first finger. Rest the backs of your wrists on your knees.

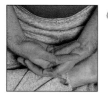

CUPPED
You can relax both hands in your lap, palms upward, one on top of the other.

CLASPED
You may also clasp your hands gently and lay them in your lap as you meditate.

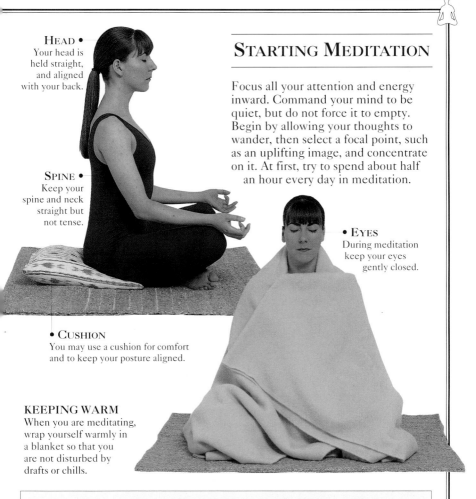

HEAD •
Your head is
held straight,
and aligned
with your back.

SPINE •
Keep your
spine and neck
straight but
not tense.

STARTING MEDITATION

Focus all your attention and energy
inward. Command your mind to be
quiet, but do not force it to empty.
Begin by allowing your thoughts to
wander, then select a focal point, such
as an uplifting image, and concentrate
on it. At first, try to spend about half
an hour every day in meditation.

• **EYES**
During meditation
keep your eyes
gently closed.

• **CUSHION**
You may use a cushion for comfort
and to keep your posture aligned.

KEEPING WARM
When you are meditating,
wrap yourself warmly in
a blanket so that you
are not disturbed by
drafts or chills.

POINTS TO REMEMBER

• Always use the same time and place to
meditate. This conditions your mind to
become calm quickly. Set aside a special
area. Do not let anything disturb you. At
first, try to sit for 20-30 minutes daily.
• Start with 5 minutes of deep abdominal
breathing. Then breathe gently, inhaling
for 3 seconds and exhaling for 3 seconds.
• You may use a **chakra** as a focal point.
If you have a rational nature, use the Ajna
Chakra, between the eyebrows. If you are
more emotional, use the Anahata Chakra,
near the heart. Never change your chakra.
• You may use a **mantra**. Repeat it once as
you inhale and once as you exhale. If you
do not have a personal mantra, use **OM**.

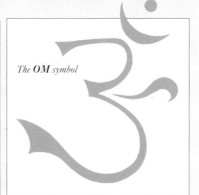

The **OM** *symbol*

HEALTH & LIFE

How the practice of yoga can aid some common ailments

·

IN ADDITION TO improving physical strength and flexibility, yoga can be helpful for those who suffer from specific complaints. While it is not regarded as a cure for physical or medical conditions, yoga can relieve many of them. Even for the fittest people, gentle physical exercise, combined with a healthy diet, can be very beneficial.

Meditation calms your mind

FOR YOUR HEALTH

Shown here are some yoga exercises that can help to relieve mental or physical problems. While these may be focused on, a full routine of **asanas** is suggested to keep the body strong and balanced.

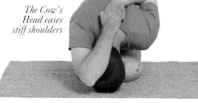

The Cow's Head eases stiff shoulders

STRESS
Asanas make your body more flexible, and release tension. **Meditation** and breathing techniques also help to lower stress levels.

ASTHMA
Backward bending exercises such as the Fish relieve congestion in your chest, and breathing exercises can help to strengthen your respiratory system.

ARTHRITIS
Arthritis sufferers may find that focusing on the Cow's Head and the sitting cycle eases stiffness in the hips and shoulders.

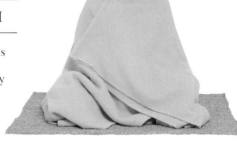

The Fish opens up your chest

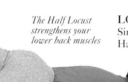

The Half Locust strengthens your lower back muscles

LOWER BACK PAIN
Single and double leg raises, and the Half Locust, will help to strengthen the muscles in your abdomen and your **lumbar** region. The Cobra and the Bow are also helpful, as they increase the flexibility of muscles in these areas.

PROPER POSTURE

Yoga promotes good posture, which relieves strain on your spine as well as improving your appearance. Imagine a line passing through the side of your body. If you are standing straight, your limbs, head, and **vertebrae** will be in alignment with this line. The images on the right show ideal posture.

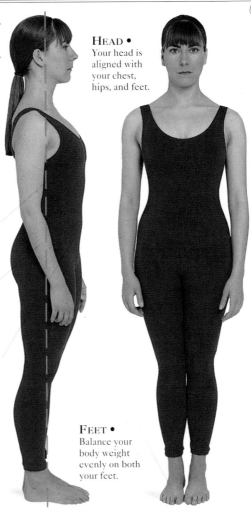

HEAD •
Your head is aligned with your chest, hips, and feet.

CHEST •
Your chest is pulled upward and does not bow in or out.

ARMS •
Let your arms hang loosely by your sides.

ABDOMEN •
Your abdomen is flat and pulled in.

LEGS AND FEET •
The line passes behind your knee joint and through your foot.

FEET •
Balance your body weight evenly on both your feet.

SPINAL STRUCTURE

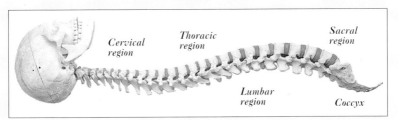

Cervical region

Thoracic region

Sacral region

Lumbar region

Coccyx

The spine has 26 **vertebrae**. At the neck are the 7 **cervical** vertebrae. Extending from the shoulders to the waist are the 12 thoracic vertebrae. The lower part of the spine contains the 5 **lumbar** vertebrae, the 5 **sacral** vertebrae, and the **coccyx**.

YOGA FOR ALL

Yoga exercises for every stage of life

WHATEVER YOUR AGE, yoga can enhance your lifestyle. For instance, it can help teenagers to keep their youthful flexibility and give them the inner strength to say no to negative influences. Older people often find that gentle yoga exercises allow them to retain mobility, and may relieve problems such as arthritis and poor circulation. Everyone can benefit from following a regular yoga routine, as it counteracts many of the problems suffered in modern life. **Asanas** release the physical tensions caused by hours of sitting, **pranayama** gives vitality by increasing the supply of oxygen to the brain, and **meditation** enhances the powers of concentration. Yoga improves strength and flexibility in the mind as well as the body, and aids relaxation. It frees the practitioner both physically and mentally, often heightening intuition and creativity.

LATER YEARS

The gentle movements used in yoga are perfectly suited to older people, especially those with an interest in physical, mental, and spiritual growth. Regular practice allows elderly people to maintain their health and mobility. Yoga can enable one to relax fully, and promotes sound sleep; it also improves digestion, stimulates circulation, and eases arthritis.

FEET •
Gentle yoga exercises
improve circulation in
your feet and hands.

• HIPS
Stiffness in your
hips can be relieved
by some **asanas**.

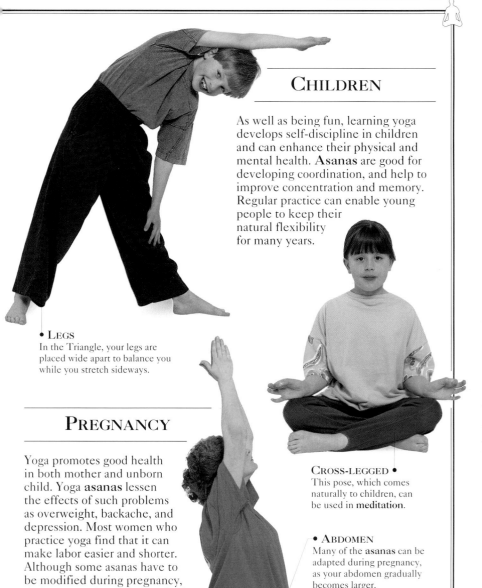

CHILDREN

As well as being fun, learning yoga develops self-discipline in children and can enhance their physical and mental health. **Asanas** are good for developing coordination, and help to improve concentration and memory. Regular practice can enable young people to keep their natural flexibility for many years.

• **LEGS**
In the Triangle, your legs are placed wide apart to balance you while you stretch sideways.

PREGNANCY

Yoga promotes good health in both mother and unborn child. Yoga **asanas** lessen the effects of such problems as overweight, backache, and depression. Most women who practice yoga find that it can make labor easier and shorter. Although some asanas have to be modified during pregnancy, their essence is perfectly suited to this time of expanded self-awareness. Pregnancy is also a very good time for **meditation**.

CROSS-LEGGED •
This pose, which comes naturally to children, can be used in **meditation**.

• **ABDOMEN**
Many of the **asanas** can be adapted during pregnancy, as your abdomen gradually becomes larger.

YOGA & SPORT

How the practice of yoga can help other sporting interests

WHATEVER SPORT you choose to practice, yoga can enhance and complement your ability. Most sports build muscular strength and stamina, often in specific areas of the body. Yoga can help to check any imbalance in muscular development, and will enable both your body and your mind to function more efficiently. If your body is flexible and supple you will be less prone to sports injuries, as your joints will be kept lubricated. Although you can focus on particular poses to help you in your chosen sport, it is always more beneficial if you complete a whole **asana** session.

LIMBS •
Yoga makes your limbs balanced, strong, and relaxed.

GOLF
Golfers may be prone to one-sided or uneven muscle development. Yoga **asanas** can strengthen weak areas and ease muscular tension.

LEGS •
The standing poses improve balance and muscle flexibility.

SKIING
Skiing demands mental alertness as well as good balance. **Asana** cycles strengthen your muscles, release physical tension, and improve your concentration and poise.

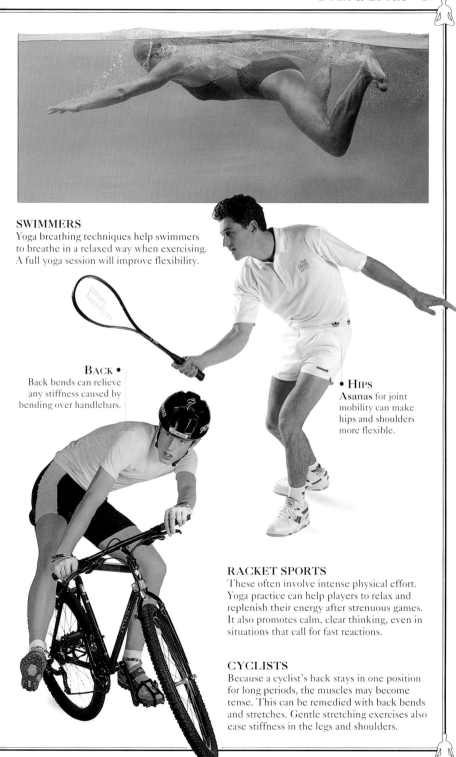

SWIMMERS
Yoga breathing techniques help swimmers to breathe in a relaxed way when exercising. A full yoga session will improve flexibility.

BACK •
Back bends can relieve any stiffness caused by bending over handlebars.

• HIPS
Asanas for joint mobility can make hips and shoulders more flexible.

RACKET SPORTS
These often involve intense physical effort. Yoga practice can help players to relax and replenish their energy after strenuous games. It also promotes calm, clear thinking, even in situations that call for fast reactions.

CYCLISTS
Because a cyclist's back stays in one position for long periods, the muscles may become tense. This can be remedied with back bends and stretches. Gentle stretching exercises also ease stiffness in the legs and shoulders.

WHERE TO PRACTICE

*Stimulating and inspirational environments for your **asanas***

•

TO VARY YOUR YOGA PRACTICE, it is sometimes helpful to give your mind a break from daily routine. Once you have mastered the skills covered in this book, you may want to practice in more congenial environments. Imagine spending a weekend, or a week, away from it all on a secluded beach or mountain top. Your day may begin with morning **meditation**, followed by **pranayama** and an **asana** session to invigorate your body. A diet of simple, nutritious foods will relax and strengthen you. If you go through your yoga routine in such peaceful surroundings, you may come to feel that you are in harmony with your inner self, humanity, and nature.

IN THE OPEN

Your yoga session can be done in any surroundings. However, as yoga is meant to balance your body and mind, it is best practiced in a natural setting where there is very little activity.

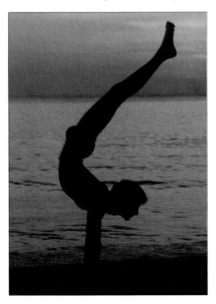

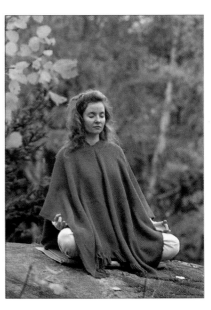

MEDITATION IN A FOREST
Being in an unspoilt place such as a forest, at a peaceful time such as sunrise, can make **meditation** easier and more meaningful.

SUNSET ON A BEACH
Sunset is also a time of peace. Practicing yoga then, surrounded by the calm and beauty of the ocean shore, can be highly beneficial.

ASHRAMS

An **ashram** is a special place set up for the teaching and daily practice of yoga. Such an environment can be a haven from the demands of everyday life, a place where you can **meditate**, relax, learn, exercise, and contact the peaceful center within yourself. A stay at an ashram will give you a taste of the healthy, balanced lifestyle that can be achieved if you follow the Five Principles of Yoga, which are given on pp.10-11: proper exercise, breathing, relaxation, diet, and positive thought and meditation. Spending time at an ashram will give your life and your practice a boost. Here you will be provided with extra encouragement and energy, and this will help you afterwards when you continue with your daily yoga sessions.

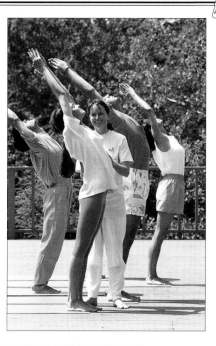

COMMUNITY SPIRIT
Doing yoga exercises in a group, such as this one at the Sivananda **Ashram** Yoga Camp in Quebec, helps to develop community spirit.

PROPER INSTRUCTION
Proper instruction is important, as can be seen in this class at the Sivananda **Ashram** Yoga Retreat on Paradise Island, Nassau, Bahamas.

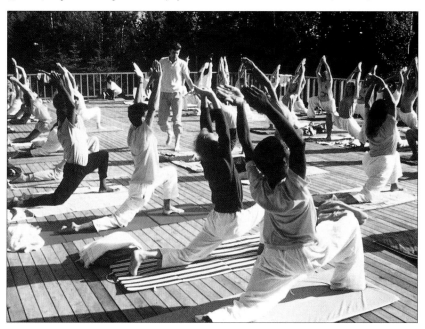

GLOSSARY

Words in *italic* are glossary entries.

A

• **Asana** A physical exercise in yoga, which is done to improve the control of body and mind. In *Sanskrit*, this word means posture, position, or seat.
• **Ashram** A peaceful retreat where yoga is taught and practiced.

C

• **Cervical vertebrae** The top 7 *vertebrae* of the spine. These bones support your neck. By holding your head correctly, you maintain their natural curvature.
• **Chakras** The 7 centers of spiritual energy in the body. The highest chakra corresponds to the pineal gland, at the top of the head, and the others lie on a line corresponding to the spinal cord.
• **Child's Pose** A relaxation pose done before and after the Headstand, and between other *asanas*. In this pose you kneel, then bend forward so that your head rests on the ground.
• **Chin Mudra** See *Mudra*.
• **Coccyx** The small curved bone at the base of the spinal column.
• **Corpse Pose** The primary relaxation pose, this is done between *asanas* and at the end of a session. Usually you lie on your back, but during the back bending cycle the Corpse can be done while lying face down.

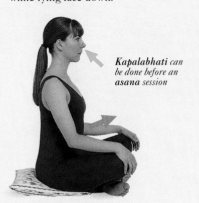

Kapalabhati can be done before an asana session

D

• **Diaphragm** The muscular partition between your lungs and your abdomen.

E

• **Easy Pose** A simple cross-legged pose that is used during warm-ups, *meditation*, and breathing exercises.

H

• **Hatha yoga** The word Hatha comes from the *Sanskrit* names for the sun and the moon, and indicates the union of opposites. Hatha yoga is the path of yoga that deals with the control of the body. The basics of this discipline are set out in the ancient scripture known as Hatha Yoga Pradipika. This work is said to have been written by the sage Swatmarama, as an inspiration from *Siva*, the first teacher of yoga.

K

• **Kapalabhati** An exercise involving rapid abdominal breathing, which is carried out to cleanse the respiratory tract. This is one of the 6 kriyas, or cleansing exercises.

L

• **Lumbar vertebrae** The lumbar group, in your lower back, consists of 5 *vertebrae*, and supports most of your body weight. This part of the spine is quite flexible. It takes on a slightly curved shape when you are standing upright or walking.

M

• **Mantra** A syllable, word, or phrase that is used to focus the mind during *meditation*. It is repeated either in your mind or aloud. The best known mantra is the syllable *Om*.
• **Meditation** A state of consciousness characterized by stillness and inner calm. The ultimate goal, in this practice, is the attainment of supreme spiritual peace.
• **Mudra** A hand position that allows the *prana* to be channelled in specific

directions. The hand positions that are featured in this book are *Chin Mudra* and *Vishnu Mudra*.

O

• **OM** This sacred syllable, sometimes written AUM, is the original *mantra*. The *Sanskrit* letter represents the journey of the human spirit toward eternal peace.

P

• **Prana** The vital energy or life force. It flows through the body along canals that are known as nadis.

• **Pranayama** Yogic breathing exercises designed for cleansing the body. In the more advanced stages, pranayama enables the practitioner to control the flow of *prana*, or vital energy, in the body.

R

• **Rajasic** The term that is used for overstimulating foods such as coffee and hot spices. These are governed by Rajas, the quality of nature that is active and restless. Rajasic foods are best avoided, as they put excessive stress on your body and mind.

S

• **Sacral vertebrae** These 5 *vertebrae* make up the lowest region of the spine. They are fused to form a single bone, which is part of the pelvic girdle.

• **Sanskrit** An ancient literary language of India.

• **Sattvic** A term used for the most wholesome foods. These are governed by Sattva, the quality of nature that is pure. Yoga practitioners usually keep to a sattvic diet, as this cleanses and invigorates the body and mind.

• **Siva** The divine inspiration for yoga. Most of the classical works on yoga are in the form of an exposition by Siva, the great yogi, to his wife Parvati.

• **Solar plexus** The network of nerves that lies just behind the stomach.

• **Sympathetic nervous system** This is part of the autonomic nervous system, which controls all involuntary muscle movements. It activates whole groups of muscles at once, in response to stimuli such as fear or excitement.

T

• **Tamasic** The word for overripe or stale foods. These are governed by Tamas, the quality of nature that is inert, and should be avoided as they cause lethargy and mental dullness.

• **Thoracic vertebrae** These are the 12 *vertebrae* in the chest area, to which the ribs are connected. This part of the spine tends to be rather rigid.

U

• **Upanishads** The ancient *Sanskrit* scriptures containing the central tenets of Hindu mysticism and philosophy.

V

• **Vedanta** The philosophy on which yoga theory is based.

• **Vertebrae** The 29 bones that form the spinal column.

• **Vishnu Mudra** See *Mudra*.

FURTHER READING

The Book of Yoga, Sivananda Yoga Center, Ebury Press
The Complete Illustrated Book of Yoga, Swami Vishnu-devananda, Harmony Books
Hatha Yoga Pradipika with Commentary Swami Vishnu-devananda, Om Lotus Publishing
Science of Pranayama, Swami Sivananda, Divine Life Society
Sivananda Yoga Video with Training Manual, Sivananda Yoga Center
Yoga Asanas, Swami Sivananda, Divine Life Society

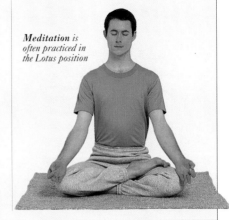

Meditation is often practiced in the Lotus position

INDEX

A

abdomen
  breathing 19
posture 85
abdominal muscles
  testing for strength 16
  in leg raises 32
Advanced Locust 53
Advanced Peacock 65
Ajna Chakra 83
alternate nostril breathing 20-21, 76
Anahata Chakra 83
arms:
  posture 85
  in relaxation 73
arthritis 84, 86
asanas
  advanced 78-9
  done outdoors 90-91
  sequence 22-3
ashrams 91
asthma 84

B

back
  back bends 54-7
  lower back pain 84
  posture 85
  stiffness 17
balancing poses 62-5
blanket
  on floor 9, 12
  in meditation 83
  in relaxation 12
body, structure 14-15
bones 15
brain, oxygen supply 86
bread 81
breathing
  alternate nostril see
    alternate nostril
    breathing
  clavicular 19
  Kapalabhati 21, 76
  meditation 82, 83
  pranayama 8, 10

relaxation 73
  single nostril 20
bronchial tubes 18, 44
Butterfly 49
buttocks, relaxation 72

C

carbohydrates 80
chakras 83
cheese 81
chest
  in Fish 44
  in relaxation 72
  posture 85
  relieving stiffness 58
children 87
Child's Pose 34
Chin Mudra 82
circulation
  in Headstand 34
  in older people 86
  in Scorpion 78
  in Shoulderstand 38
circulatory problems 86
clothes 12-13
coccyx 85
concentration
  in children 87
  in meditation 83
  in Peacock 65
  in standing poses 70-71
Corpse Pose 26, 72-3
  frontal Corpse 54
Crescent Moon 79
cushions 12, 20
cycling 89

D

Diamond 57
diaphragm 18, 19
diet 11, 80-81
Dolphin 35
double leg raise 33

E

Easy Pose 26, 27

in meditation 82
elderly people 86
eyes
  exercises 27
  in meditation 83
  in relaxation 73

F

face, relaxation 73
feet
  posture 85
  relaxation 72
Five Principles of Yoga 10-11, 91
flexibility 17
food 11, 80-81
forearms, in balancing poses 62-63
Frog 59, 77
fruit 81
Full Wheel 56, 77

G

golf 88

H

half headstand 36
Half Locust 52, 77, 84
Half Lotus 49
Half Wheel 56, 77
hamstrings 17
hands
  in meditation 82
  relaxation 73
hatha yoga 10
head
  in meditation 83
  posture 85
  relaxation 73
health 84
hips
  relaxation 72
  stiffness 86

I

illness 84
Inclined Plane 46-7, 77

insomnia 73
intercostal muscles
15, 18

J
joints
mobility 14, 58-9

K
Kapalabhati 21, 76

L
legs
leg raises 32-3, 76
posture 85
in relaxation 72
in sitting poses 48-9
in spinal twists 61
stretching 33
leotards 13
Lotus Pose 49
Fish in Lotus 45
Peacock in Lotus 79
lumbar muscles
17, 32, 84
stretching, in bridge 41
lumbar vertebrae 85

M
mantras 83
meditation 11, 82-3,
84, 86
outdoors 90
mind
in balancing poses 62
during meditation 82-3
during relaxation 73
muscles 14-15
contraction 14
extension 14
flexibility 17
in sport 88-9
relaxation 72-3
strength 16

N
neck
neck rolls 27
relieving stiffness 58
nostrils 20-21
nuts 81

O
older people 86
OM 83

P
pain, lower back 84
palming, eyes 27
Pigeon 78
positive thought 11
posture 85
practice sessions 76-7
prana 82
pranayama 8, 10,
18-21, 86
outdoors 90
Prayer Pose 28
pregnancy 87
protein 81
pulses 81

R
racket sports 89
Rajasic foods 81
relaxation 72-3, 76
benefits 10
in Child's Pose 34
in Corpse Pose
26, 72-3
Rocking Bow 55
rugs 12

S
Sattvic foods 81
Scorpion 78
seeds 81
shoulders
stiffness 44
tension 84
shoulder cycle 38-43
single leg raises 32
single nostril breathing
see breathing
sitting poses 48-9, 77
for breathing exercises
20
cross-legged 87
for meditation 82
Siva 70
skeleton 15
skiing 88
sleep 73, 86

solar plexus 10
spine 85
sport 88-9
standing asanas 66-71, 77
Hands-to-Feet Pose
66, 77
Triangle 67, 77
Triangle variations
68-9
stiffness
in the morning 9
stress 84
stretching:
muscles 16-17
stretching back 50-53
Sun Salutation 28-31, 76
swimming 89

T
T-shirts 13
Tamasic foods 81
teenagers 86
tension, in shoulders
58-9, 84
thyroid gland 38
Tortoise 79
towel, in Cow's Head 58
trachea 18
trousers 13
twists, spinal 60-61

U
Upanishads 10

V
Vedanta 10
vegetables 80
vertebrae 85
cervical 40, 44, 85
lumbar 41, 84, 85
sacral 85
thoracic 41, 85
Vishnu Mudra 20-21

W
warmth 13, 83
Warrior 59
Wheel Poses 56-7, 77
wind relieving 33

GETTING IN TOUCH

SIVANANDA YOGA
VEDANTA CENTER
243 W. 24th St.
New York, NY 10011
(212) 255-4560

SIVANANDA YOGA
VEDANTA CENTER
1600 Sawtelle Blvd.
Suite 14
Los Angeles, CA 90025

ACKNOWLEDGMENTS

The Sivananda Yoga Vedanta Center and Dorling Kindersley would
like to thank the following for their valuable help and expertise in
the production of this book:

Natalie Leucks and Shaun Mould for their tireless modeling.
Joan Butler, Leonard Gonnella, Michael Howard, Rachel Harris,
and Fiona Evans (and baby) for modeling on "Yoga for All".

Janos Marffy for all artworks and illustrations. Lol Henderson for
editorial help, and Maria D'Orsi for design assistance.
Liz Wheeler for information on anatomy and medical matters,
and Hilary Bird for the index.

Richard Bucknall for photographic assistance, and Frances Prescott
for hair styling and make-up.

Dancia International, Gamba, and Splitz for clothing. Nice Irmas for
the use of rugs and cushions. Joanne Goff for last-minute alterations.

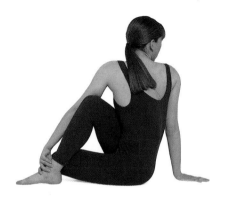